SBAs and MCQs for Drugs in Anaesthesia and Intensive Care

SBAs and MCQs for Drugs in Anaesthesia and Intensive Care

Edited by

Dr Edward Scarth

Consultant in Anaesthesia & Intensive Care Medicine
Torbay & South Devon NHS Foundation Trust
Torbay Hospital, UK

Dr Claire Blandford

Consultant Anaesthetist
Torbay & South Devon NHS Foundation Trust
Torbay Hospital, UK;
and Clinical Subdean
University of Exeter Medical School
Exeter, UK

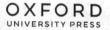

OXFORD
UNIVERSITY PRESS

OXFORD
UNIVERSITY PRESS

Great Clarendon Street, Oxford, OX2 6DP,
United Kingdom

Oxford University Press is a department of the University of Oxford.
It furthers the University's objective of excellence in research, scholarship,
and education by publishing worldwide. Oxford is a registered trade mark of
Oxford University Press in the UK and in certain other countries

Published in the United States of America by Oxford University Press
198 Madison Avenue, New York, NY 10016, United States of America

British Library Cataloguing in Publication Data

Data available

Library of Congress Control Number: 2022945863

ISBN 978-0-19-882698-9

DOI: 10.1093/med/9780198826989.001.0001

Printed in the UK by
Ashford Colour Press Ltd, Gosport, Hampshire

Foreword

An in-depth understanding of pharmacology is essential within anaesthetic and intensive care medical practice. However, it is an area that many trainees preparing for exams (and indeed more experienced colleagues) find particularly challenging. This exam preparation book is an excellent companion to the already well-recognized publication *Drugs in Anaesthesia and Intensive Care*.

The authors draw on an impressive range of experience in this field, Dr Scarth having co-authored the fourth and fifth editions of the companion text and Dr Blandford having established and run for many years the extremely successful South West Intensive Primary Examination day (SWIPED) with accompanying published Structured Oral Examination (SOE) exam preparation text (*Passing the Primary FRCA SOE*).

The chapters are arranged to cover all the main pharmacological topics required within anaesthetic/intensive care practice and a wide range of both multiple-choice and single best answer questions ensure that a candidate will be fully prepared to tackle the finer details of the pharmacology syllabuses of these professional examinations. I imagine that this book will prove invaluable to both trainees and trainers, and both will be more fully educated in the finer points of pharmacology after working through these questions together!

Dr Mary Stocker MA Chemistry (Oxon), *MBChB, FRCA*
Consultant Anaesthetist, *Torbay and South Devon*

Preface

This book has been a collaboration between two consultant colleagues at Torbay & South Devon NHS Foundation Trust. Drs Blandford and Scarth have almost 40 years of combined experience in the field of anaesthetics and intensive care medicine.

Dr Blandford is a consultant anaesthetist with clinical interests in orthopaedics, regional anaesthesia, day surgery, and clinical pathway quality improvement. She has a strong educational background, having established and led as course director a well-respected national exam preparation course for the primary FRCA examination for over a decade and published her first educational text in 2016, *Passing the Primary FRCA SOE—A Practical Guide*. Dr Blandford continues to support trainees as an educational supervisor, IAC programme lead for her department, and since 2019 has been a Clinical Subdean for the University of Exeter Medical School, jointly holding the position of Director of Undergraduate Medical Education at her trust.

Dr Scarth is a consultant in Anaesthesia and Intensive Care Medicine. He has clinical interests that include the transfer of critically ill patients and has previously supported the regional transfer medicine service as a consultant coordinator. He also has clinical experience in delayed primary and secondary aeromedical retrieval medicine. Dr Scarth holds a senior clinical governance position in the trust's management structure and is responsible for overseeing governance across numerous clinical departments. He has an interest in incident investigation and patient safety. In 2016 Dr Scarth co-authored the revised 5th edition of the much-respected pharmacology book, *Drugs in Anaesthesia and Intensive Care*, which I'm sure most of us (both authors included!) had an edition of on the pile of revision resources when examinations came around.

This new book is designed as a companion to *Drugs in Anaesthesia and Intensive Care*, however, it can also be used as a standalone preparation text. Pharmacology is often an area of examination syllabuses in which learners struggle. The breadth of the topics covered and the detail within which questions may be asked is frequently daunting. This book acts as a dedicated pharmacology resource to help you hone your learning and examination practice. It has been designed to cover multiple syllabuses across the anaesthesia and intensive care postgraduate examinations offering an adaptable resource for your preparation.

We both wish you well in your examination success and hope this book helps you along the way.

Dr Claire Blandford
Dr Edward Scarth Torbay
May 2022

Contents

Abbreviations

ADH	Antidiuretic hormone
AKI	Acute kidney injury
AMPK	Adenosine monophosphate kinase
ARDS	Acute respiratory distress syndrome
ATD	Adult therapeutic dose
CK	Creatinine kinase
CKD	Chronic kidney disease
CMR	Cerebral metabolic rate
CNS	Central nervous system
CPP	Cerebral perfusion pressure
CRS	Cytokine-release syndrome
DI	Diabetes insipidus
ED	Effective dosages
ED	Emergency department
EDAIC	European Diploma in Anaesthesiology and Intensive Care
EDIC	European Diploma in Intensive Care
FFICM	Fellowship of the Faculty of Intensive Care Medicine
FFP	Fresh frozen plasma
FRC	Functional residual capacity
FRCA	Fellowship of the Royal College of Anaesthetists
GCS	Glasgow Coma Scale
GvHD	Graft versus host disease
HAS	Human albumin solution
ICU	Intensive care unit
LVOT	Left ventricular outflow tract
MAP	Mean arterial pressure
MCQ	Multiple-Choice Questions
MH	Malignant hypertermia
NMDA	N-methyl D-aspartate
PABA	Para-amino benzoic acid
PAS	Platelet additive solution
PBPC	Peripheral blood progenitor cells
PEP	Post-exposure prophylaxis
PPI	Proton pump inhibitor

PSE	Present State Examination
PUD	Peptic ulcer disease
RBC	Red blood cell
RRT	Renal replacement therapy
RSI	Rapid sequence induction
SBA	Single Best Answer
SCRA	Synthetic cannabinoid receptor agonists
SIADH	Syndrome of inappropriate antidiuretic hormone
SSRI	Selective serotonin reuptake inhibitors
SVP	Saturated vapour pressure
SVR	Systemic vascular resistance
TIVA	Total intravenous anaesthesia
TLS	Tumour lysis syndrome
TOF	Train-of-four
VD	Volume of distribution

Contributors

Dr Claire Blandford
Consultant Anaesthetist, Torbay
& South Devon NHS Foundation
Trust, Torbay Hospital, UK; and
Clinical Subdean, University
of Exeter Medical School,
Exeter, UK
Chapters 1, 3, 6

Dr David Hutchins
Consultant in Anaesthesia
and Pain Medicine, University
Hospitals Plymouth,
Plymouth, UK
Chapter 6 co-author

Dr David Levy
Consultant Anaesthetist, Torbay
& South Devon NHS Foundation
Trust, Torbay Hospital, UK
Chapters 2, 10, 15

Dr Graham C. McCracken
Registrar in Intensive Care
Medicine and Anaesthesia, Belfast
Health and Social Care Trust,
Northern Ireland, UK
Chapters 4, 9, 13

Dr Helen Marshall
Consultant Anaesthetist, Royal
Devon University Hospital
(Eastern), NHS Foundation
Trust, Exeter, UK
Chapters 11, 12, 14

Dr Sarah Shaw
Anaesthetic Registrar, Torbay &
South Devon NHS Foundation
Trust, Torbay Hospital,
Torquay, UK
Chapters 5, 8

Dr Edward Scarth
Consultant in Anaesthesia &
Intensive Care Medicine, Torbay
& South Devon NHS Foundation
Trust, Torbay Hospital, UK
Chapters 7, 16, 17

Chapter 1

Inhaled anaesthetic agents

QUESTIONS

Multiple-Choice Questions

1. Which of the following statements are true?

A The potency of an inhaled anaesthetic agent can be indicated by its blood:gas partition coefficient

B A high oil:gas partition coefficient indicates an inhaled anaesthetic agent with a rapid onset/offset time

C An 'ideal' volatile anaesthetic agent would have a high oil:gas coefficient value and a low blood:gas coefficient value

D Pyrexia lowers the blood:gas coefficient value of sevoflurane

E MAC_{bar} is the brain concentration of an anaesthetic agent which blocks adrenergic responses to a standardized skin incision in 50% of patients

2. Regarding xenon:

A Xenon has a high blood:gas partition coefficient

B Xenon is an odourless gas

C Xenon inhibits $GABA_A$ receptors

D Xenon is a potent analgesic

E Xenon is contraindicated in patients with malignant hyperpyrexia

3. Which of the following drugs are correctly matched with their chemical formulae?

A Desflurane = $C_3H_2F_6O$

B Enflurane = $C_3H_2ClF_5O$

C Halothane = $C_4H_3F_7O$

D Isoflurane = $C_3H_2BrF_5O$

E Sevoflurane = $C_2H_3ClF_7O$

4. Concerning methoxyflurane, which of the following are true?

A Concerns about hepatic toxicity led to it being withdrawn from the UK

B When used as an anaesthetic, an analgesic effect persists into the postoperative period

C Onset time is rapid

D Has a higher incidence of dysrhythmia than halothane

E Has no effect on APGAR scores when used in labour

5. Heliox

A Is a mixture of 50% He: 50% O_2

B Heliox cylinders are green with white shoulders in the UK

C Has approximately 33% of the density of air

D Has approximately the same viscosity as air

E Is approved as a definitive treatment for acute severe asthma

6. Which of the following statements concerning inhalational anaesthetics are true?

A Desflurane has been shown experimentally to enhance activity of pre- and postsynaptic 'two-pore domain potassium channels'

B Volatile anaesthetic agents prolong the $GABA_A$ receptor-mediated excitatory chloride ion current

C Nitrous oxide has an inhibitory action at N-methyl-D-aspartate (NMDA) receptors

D Volatile anaesthetic agents are agonists at neuronal glutamate receptors

E Volatile anaesthetic agents are antagonists at neuronal glycine receptors

7. When inducing anaesthesia with volatile agents, which of the following statements are true?

A A large functional residual capacity (FRC) results in faster onset of anaesthesia

B A lower breathing system volume increases the F_A/F_i ratio

C Lower levels of albumin may contribute to a more rapid onset of volatile anaesthesia

D The 'second gas effect' of nitrous oxide reduces the alveolar partial pressures of co-administered volatile agents during induction

E Increasing haematocrit increases the solubility of enflurane

Single Best Answers

1. Bloods taken from a 62-year-old female patient a week following spinal surgery showed macrocytic anaemia and an elevated plasma homocysteine level. Preoperatively results were all within normal limits. Which one of the following is most likely to be associated with these findings?

A Desflurane

B Isoflurane

C Nitrous oxide

D Oxygen

E Sevoflurane

2. A new inhaled anaesthetic drug 'R' has been discovered. You are told the following information:

```
Molecular weight = 144
Boiling point = 49°C
Blood:Gas partition coefficient = 0.20
Oil:Gas partition coefficient = 150
MAC = 0.9
```

Which statement is most likely to be true about this drug?

A Drug 'R' is a structural isomer of sevoflurane

B Drug 'R' is less potent than isoflurane

C Drug 'R' is likely to require a vaporizer similar in design to a desflurane vaporizer

D Drug 'R' will have a faster rate of onset than desflurane

E Drug 'R' would be expected to have a MAC_{aw} value of 0.1

3. A 21-year primigravida has laboured to 9 cm cervical dilatation. She now requires general anaesthesia for an emergency caesarean section due to profound foetal bradycardia. Which of the following gas mixtures would you expect to result in the least intraoperative blood loss?

A 29% Oxygen/70% nitrous oxide/0.8% isoflurane

B 40% Oxygen/57% medical air/3% isoflurane

C 45% Oxygen/50% medical air/5% sevoflurane

D 60% Oxygen/38% nitrous oxide/1.5% isoflurane

E 96% Oxygen/4% isoflurane

4. A 20-year-old ASA 1 man is undergoing the removal of metal work from his ankle. His general anaesthetic was induced with propofol, fentanyl, and atracurium. He is intubated and ventilated with a gas mixture comprising oxygen, medical air, and sevoflurane. Approximately 30 minutes into the case, tachycardia and a substantial rise in end-tidal carbon dioxide are noted. This patient has had two previous uneventful general anaesthetics.

Which of the following drugs is likely to be the most useful in this patient's management?

A Adrenaline 1:1000

B Cyproheptadine

C Dantrolene

D Phentolamine

E Propylthiouracil

5. You are given the following data about an inhaled anaesthetic agent:

```
Saturated vapour pressure (SVP) at 20°C: 32 kPa
Blood:gas partition coefficient: 1.40
Oil:gas partition coefficient: 97
```

Which of the following is this agent most likely to be?

A Desflurane

B Enflurane

C Halothane

D Isoflurane

E Sevoflurane

6. Seven days post surgery, a 50-year-old woman develops pyrexia, non specific gastrointestinal upset and a rash. An eosinophilia is noted on her full blood count. Which drug is she most likely to have been exposed to that could account for these symptoms?

A Desflurane

B Enflurane

C Halothane

D Methoxyflurane

E Nitrous oxide

7. A 50-year-old man is having an inhalational anaesthetic at 3000 m altitude. Which statement about the conduct of his anaesthetic is most accurate:

A At this altitude the dial on an isoflurane vaporizer should be set to half of the desired 'sea level' % setting

B A sevoflurane vaporizer set to 4% will produce a partial pressure of 70% of its 'sea level' value

C A Tec-6 desflurane vaporizer can be used at this altitude with no compensation required for atmospheric pressure changes due to its design features

D Setting the dial on an isoflurane vaporizer to 1% will produce the same partial pressure at this altitude as it would at sea level

E The SVP of a volatile agent is reduced by low ambient pressure

ANSWERS

Multiple-Choice Questions

1. FFTTT

Potency of anaesthetic agents is associated with the oil:gas partition coefficient, not the blood:gas partition coefficient. The oil:gas coefficient increases as the potency of an agent increases. The blood:gas partition coefficient is a measure of the agent's solubility. A high blood:gas solubility value means a greater amount is taken up in the blood and it takes longer for partial pressure equilibrium to be reached, thus induction times will be slower.

An 'ideal' volatile anaesthetic agent would therefore have a high oil:gas coefficient value (for potency) and a low blood:gas coefficient value (for speed of induction). Pyrexia reduces the blood:gas coefficients of inhaled anaesthetic agents, which typically makes induction in hyperthermic patients more rapid.

MAC defines the minimum alveolar concentration of anaesthetic gas at 1 atmosphere required to prevent a movement response in 50% of subjects undergoing a standard surgical stimulus. Its units are percentages. MAC_{bar} uses changes in heart rate and arterial pressure as indicators of adrenergic responses to incision. Values are presented as fractions of MAC. Opiates significantly reduce MAC_{bar} values but have a ceiling of effect.

Further reading

Charlton M, Thompson JP. Pharmacokinetics in sepsis. *BJA Education*, 2019;19(1):7–13.

Smith S, Scarth E. *Drugs in Anaesthesia and Intensive Care*, 5th edition. Oxford University Press, 2016. APPENDIX A1.1.

White D. Uses of MAC. *Br J Anaesth*, 2003;91(2):167–169.

2. FTFTF

Xenon, a noble gas, has many advantageous anaesthetic properties. It has an extremely low blood:gas partition coefficient (0.14)—lower than all the other agents that are currently available. A low blood:gas partition coefficient is associated with rapid onset and offset of action. It is indeed an odourless gas. Xenon's mechanism of action is thought to be potent non-competitive inhibition of NMDA receptors with little effect on $GABA_A$ receptors. Xenon does indeed have a potent analgesic effect, it is thought to be superior to nitrous oxide in this property. Nitrous oxide promotes release of endogenous ligands for opiate receptors, yet the mechanism for xenon is thought to be antinociceptive at a spinal cord level. *In-vivo* and *in-vitro* studies indicate that xenon is not a trigger for malignant hyperpyrexia in susceptible individuals.

Further reading

Sanders RD, Franks NP, Maze M. Xenon: no stranger to anaesthesia. *Br J Anaesth*, 2003;91(5):709–717.

Smith S, Scarth E. Drugs in Anaesthesia *and* Intensive Care, 5th edition. Oxford University Press, 2016. Nitrous Oxide, Xenon.

3. TTFFF

Correct answers are:

Desflurane = $C_3H_2F_6O$
Halothane = $C_2HBrClF_3$
Isoflurane/Enflurane = $C_3H_2ClF_5O$
Sevoflurane = $C_4H_3F_7O$

Isoflurane and enflurane are structural isomers thus they have the same chemical formulae but a different spatial arrangement of atoms. Halothane is the only agent to contain bromine (which of note also makes it radio-opaque).

Further reading

Smith S, Scarth E. *Drugs in Anaesthesia and Intensive Care*, 5th edition. Oxford University Press, 2016. Desflurane, Enflurane, Halothane, Isoflurane, Sevoflurane.

4. FTTFT

Methoxyflurane is a halogenated volatile anaesthetic agent which was commonly used in the 1960s–1970s. It had a rapid time to onset, cardiovascular stability (low incidence of dysrhythmias) and particularly of interest, an analgesic effect which extended into the postanaesthetic period. Its use declined due to concerns about nephrotoxicity following deep anaesthesia with this agent and ultimately lead to it being withdrawn from the UK. There have been rare reports of hepatic toxicity but these were felt to be idiosyncratic reactions.

Methoxyflurane continued to be used at subanaesthetic doses, especially in Australia and New Zealand—exploiting its function as an inhaled analgesic agent and has now been re-registered in Europe under the brand name Penthrox® (2015). It is licenced for use in conscious adults to alleviate moderate/severe pain, especially in trauma. At subanaesthetic doses, fluoride levels are below the renal threshold of concern. It has also been used for obstetric analgesia where it has been found to be better tolerated than Entonox® and does not affect APGAR scores.

Further reading

Jephcott C, Grummet J, Nguyen N, Spruyt O. A review of the safety and efficacy of inhaled methoxyflurane as an analgesic for outpatient procedures. *Br J Anaesth*, 2018;120(5);1040–1048.

Porter KM, Dayan AD, Dickerson S, Middleton PM. The role of inhaled methoxyflurane in acute pain management. *Open Access Emerg Med*, 2018;10:149–164.

5. FFTTF

Helium is an inert gas of low molecular weight (atomic weight 4). It is presented in the UK in brown cylinders as 100% helium, or if presented as heliox (a mixture of 79% helium: 21% oxygen) the cylinders are white with brown and white shoulders. Heliox has a specific gravity of 0.337, significantly lower than either air (1) or oxygen (1.091) (for reference, the specific gravity of Helium is 0.178). It is this low specific gravity conferring low density which gives Helium its key property for medical use. The lower the density of a gas, the proportionally higher the flow rate. Heliox also assists in converting areas of turbulent flow within the bronchial tree into laminar flow by reducing Reynolds (Re) number (note: flow is predominantly laminar when Re <2000 and turbulent when Re >4000). This lowered resistance increases ventilation and reduces the work of breathing. It has been successfully used as a temporizing measure in severe asthma or other causes of airway obstruction while definitive treatment is instituted but it is not classed as a definitive treatment in its own right. Despite having a much lower density than air, heliox has a viscosity very similar to air. This is because nitrogen and helium have very similar viscosities and are present in approximately similar proportions in air and heliox, respectively.

Further reading

Reuben AD, Harris AR. Heliox for asthma in the emergency department: a review of the literature. *Emerg Med J*, 2004;21:131–135.

6. TFTFF

Two-pore domain potassium channels are found pre- and postsynpatically throughout the central nervous system. Desflurane (along with isoflurane, sevoflurane, and halothane) has been found to enhance the activity of these channels leading to membrane hyperpolarization.

Halogenated volatile anaesthetic agents prolong the $GABA_A$ receptor-mediated inhibitory chloride current whereas nitrous oxide and xenon have been found to have inhibitory actions at NMDA receptors. Volatile agents are antagonists at presynaptic excitatory glutamate receptors and agonists at inhibitory postsynaptic glycine receptors.

Further reading

Khan KS, Hayes I, Buggy DJ. Pharmacology of anaesthetic agents II: inhalation anaesthetic agents. Contin Educ Anaesth Crit Care *Pain*, 2014;14(3):106–111.

Smith S, Scarth E. *Drugs in Anaesthesia and Intensive Care*, 5th edition. Oxford University Press, 2016. Desflurane, Halothane, Isoflurane, Nitrous Oxide, Sevoflurane.

7. FTTFT

Large FRCs lead to dilution of the inspired anaesthetic agent and hence a lower alveolar partial pressure. This means there is a slower onset of anaesthesia. A breathing circuit with a lower volume will tend to have a higher inspired gas concentration, which results in more rapid increase of the alveolar concentration of agent (F_A) towards the inspired concentration (F_i) and faster speed of induction.

Lower levels of albumin (seen in children and elderly adults) reduce the blood:gas solubility coefficients of volatile agents and contribute to more rapid onset of anaesthesia. This effect is clinically seen less with sevoflurane and desflurane due to their relatively low blood:gas solubility coefficient values. The second gas effect occurs because nitrous oxide (N_2O) is 30 times more soluble than nitrogen. N_2O is rapidly taken up from the alveolus resulting in a loss of alveolar volume which relatively concentrates and increases the alveolar partial pressures of other co-administered volatile agents.

Enflurane has affinity for red blood cells so increasing haematocrit results in more enflurane binding, thus increasing its solubility as the red blood cells are acting as a binding 'sink'

Further reading

Khan KS, Hayes I, Buggy DJ. Pharmacology of anaesthetic agents II: inhalation anaesthetic agents. *Contin Educ Anaesth Crit Care Pain*, 2014;14(3):106–111.

Smith S, Scarth E. *Drugs in Anaesthesia and Intensive Care*, 5th edition. Oxford University Press, 2016. Enflurane, Nitrous Oxide, Appendix A1.1.

Single Best Answers

1. C

Megaloblastic anaemia can develop following exposure to nitrous oxide. There are many drug-induced causes of megaloblastic anaemia but of the list presented, only nitrous oxide is associated. It can occur in patients with previously normal levels of vitamin B_{12} but is more common in those with pre-existing (often undiagnosed) vitamin B_{12} deficiency and is significantly associated with duration of exposure to the agent. Nitrous oxide irreversibly oxidizes cobalamin contained within vitamin B_{12} into an inactive form. This inactive form prevents methionine synthase from converting homocysteine to form methionine (and thus leads to elevated homocysteine levels). The transmethylation reaction is essential for DNA synthesis and its absence leads to nuclear immature red blood cells being released into the circulation. Neurological deficits such as numbness, weakness, and paraesthesia can also present and in rare cases subacute combined degeneration of the cord has been diagnosed.

Further reading

Hadzic A, Glab K, Sanborn K, Thys D: severe neurological deficit after nitrous oxide anaesthesia. *Anaesthesiology*, 1995;83:863–866.

Smith S, Scarth E. *Drugs in Anaesthesia and Intensive Care*, 5th edition. Oxford University Press, 2016. Nitrous oxide.

2. D

The agent quoted has a higher oil:gas coefficient value than isoflurane (97) and thus is a more potent agent. MAC_{aw} refers to MAC_{awake}. It is typically expressed as a fraction of MAC. Studies on modern anaesthetic agents have concluded its typical value to be one-third of the MAC value of that specific agent so in the case of drug R above you would expect a value near 0.3. The blood:gas partition coefficient indicates an agent's solubility. A low value suggests a relatively insoluble gas which will rapidly achieve partial pressure equilibrium between blood and alveolar gas and thus have a rapid onset time, as the value quoted is lower than that of desflurane (0.45) and therefore it will have a faster onset/offset time than desflurane. The molecular weight is the sum of the atomic weights of the molecule's constituent atoms. Structural isomers will have identical molecular weights and as the molecular weight of sevoflurane is 200, drug 'R' cannot be a structural isomer of it.

Drug 'R' has a boiling point much higher than the UK room temperature range, so compensation beyond the conventional temperature-compensated plenum vaporizer design is unlikely to be required.

Further reading

Smith S, Scarth E. *Drugs in Anaesthesia and Intensive Care*, 5th edition. Oxford University Press, 2016. Desflurane, Isoflurane, Sevoflurane, Appendix A1.1.

White D. Uses of MAC. *Br J Anaesth*, 2003;91(2):167–169.

3. A

All volatile halogenated anaesthetic agents cause uterine relaxation (tocolysis), dilate uterine arteries, and increase uterine blood flow in a dose-related relationship. Post delivery, the re-establishment of uterine tone is a key factor which modifies the degree of blood loss, especially for a lower segment caesarean section (LSCS) performed at almost full cervical dilation. Uterine atony is one of the major causes of post-partum haemorrhage. Nitrous oxide does not cause uterine relaxation and thus its use to contribute to the necessary MAC of anaesthesia reduces the required contribution of volatile anaesthetic agent and will be associated with less uterine relaxation and less bleeding. Therefore answer 'D', which quotes the lowest volatile agent %, is the correct response.

Further reading

Smith S, Scarth E. *Drugs in Anaesthesia and Intensive Care*, 5th edition. Oxford University Press, 2016. Isoflurane, Nitrous oxide, Sevoflurane.

4. C

The diagnosis is malignant hyperthermia (MH), a hypermetabolic state triggered by volatile agents and neuromuscular blocking drugs in susceptible individuals. Clinical features include rising end-tidal carbon dioxide (or tachypnoea in the spontaneously ventilating patient), muscle rigidity, masseter spasm, pyrexia, and unexplained tachycardia. Previous uneventful anaesthesia is common. Key management includes cessation of all trigger agents, administration of dantrolene, active cooling, and supportive care. Dantrolene acts to inhibit calcium release in muscle fibres, thus uncoupling the dysregulated cellular system.

Adrenaline 1:1000 (IM) is used as part of the management of anaphylaxis (although a potential differential, the high end-tidal carbon dioxide makes MH the more likely answer). Other differentials for MH include thyroid storm, neuroleptic malignant syndrome, serotonin syndrome, and phaeochromocytoma; however, the description of the patient as ASA1 would indicate these are not likely in this scenario. For reference: cyproheptadine has been used to manage severe serotonin syndrome reactions, phentolamine is an alpha blocker, and propylthiouracil reduces the synthesis and peripheral conversion of thyroid hormones.

Further reading

Gupta PK, Hopkins PM. Diagnosis and management of malignant hyperthermia. *BJA Education*, 2017;17 (7):249–254.

Smith S, Scarth E. *Drugs in Anaesthesia and Intensive Care*, 5th edition. Oxford University Press, 2016. Adrenaline, Atracurium, Dantrolene, Fentanyl, Phentolamine, Propofol, Sevoflurane.

5. D

The data provided corresponds to isoflurane.

For comparison, see Table 1.1.

Further reading

Smith S, Scarth E. *Drugs in Anaesthesia and Intensive Care*, 5th edition. Oxford University Press, 2016. Desflurane, Enflurane, Isoflurane, Sevoflurane, Appendix A1.1.

6. C

The clinical features are descriptive of halothane hepatitis. An unexplained postoperative pyrexia is characteristically the initial presenting feature, classically occurring seven days post exposure initial exposure or earlier following multiple exposures to halothane. Other clinical features include arthralgia and jaundice. Bloods reveal eosinophilia in up to one-third of patients. Type 1 halothane hepatitis is generally mild and self-limiting. Type 2 is a severe hepatotoxicity reaction and can be fatal. Halothane use has largely been replaced by more modern agents in the developed world, yet it is still used in Africa and the Middle East.

Table 1.1 Comparison table of volatile anaesthetic agents and their pharmacochemical properties

	Sevoflurane	Desflurane	Enflurane	Halothane	Isoflurane	N₂O
MW	200	168	184.5	197.4	184.5	44
BP °C	58.6	22.8	56.5	50.2	48.5	−88.5
SVP (kPa) at 20°C	22.7	88.5	23.3	32	32	5200
MAC %	1.8	6.6	1.68	0.75	1.15	105
B:G coeff	0.7	0.45	1.91	2.5	1.4	0.47
O:G coeff	50	29	98	224	97	1.4

Key: MW = molecular weight; MAC = minimum alveolar concentration; BP = boiling point; B:G coeff = blood:gas partition coefficient; SVP = saturated vapour pressure;
O:G coeff = oil:gas partition coefficient.

Further reading

Ray DC, Drummond GB. Halothane hepatitis. *Br J Anaesth*, 1991;67:84–99.

Smith S, Scarth E. *Drugs in Anaesthesia and Intensive Care*, 5th edition. Oxford University Press, 2016. Halothane.

7. D

At 3000 m atmospheric pressure will be approx. 70 kPa (0.7bar). The SVP of an agent is unaffected by ambient pressure alone, providing temperature compensation occurs. Modern vaporizers together with environmental insulation from buildings or aircraft will be able to temperature compensate for operating at this altitude. The net effect of increasing altitude is that the output of the vaporizer actually increases but the agent's partial pressure is maintained so no additional calibration/compensation is required when using a isoflurane/sevoflurane/halothane vaporizer at altitude. The different design features of a desflurane vaporizer means that the concentration delivered is unaffected by ambient pressure and thus a reduced agent partial pressure will be produced, unless the unit is recalibrated or the dial setting appropriately adjusted.

Further reading

Boumphrey S, Marshall N. Understanding vaporizers. *Cont Educ Anaesth Crit Care Pain*, 2011;11(6):199–203.

Smith S, Scarth E. *Drugs in Anaesthesia and Intensive Care*, 5th edition. Oxford University Press, 2016. Desflurane, Halothane, Isoflurane, Sevoflurane, Appendix A1.1.

Intravenous anaesthetic agents

QUESTIONS

Multiple Choice Questions

1. Regarding ketamine:

A the R-(−) enantiomer has four times greater affinity for its receptor

B it has poor oral bioavailability

C ketamine may be administered extradurally and intrathecally

D it is highly protein bound

E metabolism produces norketamine, which is an active metabolite

2. Following a 0.3 mg/kg dose of etomidate, which of the following effects might you expect?

A analgesia

B coughing

C hypotension

D laryngospasm

E pain on injection

3. Which of the following statements regarding the following intravenous induction agents are true?

A etomidate has a large volume of distribution

B ketamine is poorly protein bound

C propofol is highly protein bound

D thiopental, in comparison to other IV agents, has the longest elimination half-life

E thiopental is highly unionized at physiological pH

4. The dose of propofol required for induction can be decreased by which of the following drugs?

A clonidine

B ephedrine

C midazolam

D ondansetron

E remifentanil

5. Regarding propofol:

A it has a hydroxyl group on its first carbon

B it contains 2.25 mg/ml glycerol

C it may be administered intramuscularly

D it should not be used in infusion in liver disease due to risk of accumulation

E it may increase the energy required for successful cardioversion

6. The following are features of propofol infusion syndrome:

A bradycardia

B convex ST elevation

C hyperlipidaemia

D hyperthermia

E myoglobinuria

7. The following drugs are incompatible when mixed:

A ketamine–propofol

B ketamine–thiopental

C propofol–suxamethonium

D thiopental–mivacurium

E thiopental–rocuronium

Single Best Answers

1. Epileptiform movements are noted during IV induction in a 52-year-old woman. Which drug is the patient most likely to have been given?

A etomidate

B ketamine

C midazolam

D propofol

E thiopental

2. A patient has been given a 2 mg/kg intravenous bolus of ketamine. Which of these clinical effects would be the most likely to occur?

A bradycardia

B bronchospasm

C decreased uterine tone

D increased gastric mobility

E salivation

3. Which of these statements is the most appropriate explanation of how etomidate administration inhibits steroidogenesis?

A inhibition of 5-α-reductase

B inhibition of aromatase

C inhibition of 3-β dehydroxysteroid dehydrogenase

D inhibition of 11-β hydroxylase

E inhibition of 21-hydroxylase

4. Which of the following factors increases potency and onset of action when compared to other barbiturates?

A a hydrogen at N1 and oxygen at C2

B a hydrogen at N1 and sulphur atom at C2

C a methyl side group at N1 and oxygen at C2

D a pair of oxygen atoms at C4 and C6

E a phenyl side chain at C5 and nitrogen atom at C2

5. What best describes the main mechanism of action of ketamine?

A antagonism of the effect of glutamate

B blockade of voltage-gated calcium channels

C γ-Aminobutyric acid (GABA) agonism

D it is a highly selective α-2 agonist

E it is a sodium channel blocker

6. Which factor makes propofol well-suited for neuroanaesthesia?

A cerebral metabolic rate (CMR) remains unchanged

B it increases cerebral perfusion pressure (CPP)

C metabolic blood flow coupling remains unchanged

D there is an increase in synaptic activity

E unchanged cerebral oxygen consumption

7. Which is the best statement explaining why thiopental is not suit-able for total intravenous anaesthesia (TIVA)?

A It has a hepatic extraction coefficient of 0.1

B It has a small volume of distribution

C It has many active metabolites

D It irreversibly binds to GABA receptors

E It is poorly lipid soluble

ANSWERS

Multiple Choice Questions

1. FTTFT

Ketamine is a phencyclidine derivative made up of equal proportions of S-(+) and R-(–) ketamine, with the cyclohexanone rings producing a chiral centre. It is available as both a racemic mixture and as the S-(+) enantiomer. S-(+) ketamine has four times greater affinity for its receptor and is three times as potent as the R-(–) form.

pH of preparations varies from 3.5 to 5.5. It is highly lipid soluble and has a pK_a of 7.5 and so is 44% unionized at physiological pH. It may be administered intravenously, intramuscularly, orally, rectally, and nasally. It can be given extradurally and intrathecally but the preservative-free preparation must be used in this case.

Bioavailability orally is 20–25%, nasally is 25–50% and intramuscularly is 93%. Ketamine is 20–50% protein bound with a volume of distribution (V_D) of 3 L/kg with recovery occurring due to redistribution of the drug. It is metabolized in the liver by N-demethylation and hydroxylation via the CYP450 system. It forms norketamine, which has 30% the activity of ketamine, which is then conjugated to form inactive metabolites.

Further reading

Hardman JG, Hopkins PM, Stuys MMRF. *Oxford Textbook of Anaesthesia*. Oxford University Press, 2017. Intravenous anaesthetics.

Smith S, Scarth E. *Drugs in Anaesthesia and Intensive Care*, 5th edition. Oxford University Press, 2016. Ketamine.

2. FTTTT

Although etomidate is traditionally thought of as the drug of cardiovascular stability for induction of general anaesthesia, it still causes a mild degree of hypotension. There may be a slight compensatory tachycardia. There is a dose-dependent reduction in respiratory rate and tidal volume. Hiccupping may accompany induction in 20% of patients and coughing and laryngospasm may occur. Pain on injection is common, occurring in 25–50% of cases. There is a 20–30% decrease in cerebral blood flow with a reduction in intracranial and intraocular pressure. It is emetogenic, and this is particularly apparent in patients also receiving opioids. Unlike ketamine, etomidate does not have intrinsic analgesic properties and the haemodynamic response to laryngoscopy will not be attenuated. Prolongation of the bleeding time may occur with its use due to its antiplatelet activity.

Further reading

Hardman JG, Hopkins PM, Stuys MMRF. *Oxford Textbook of Anaesthesia*. Oxford University Press, 2017. Intravenous anaesthetics.

Smith S, Scarth E. *Drugs in Anaesthesia and Intensive Care*, 5th edition. Oxford University Press, 2016. Etomidate.

3. TTTFT

See Table 2.1. V_D is the apparent volume that a drug distributes to achieve its final concentration. Drugs that are highly ionized and have high protein binding generally have low V_D. Albumin binds to acidic drugs, while α-1-acid glycoprotein binds to basic drugs. Protein binding has importance, in that it is the free drug that is biologically active and certain diseases or other drugs will affect this proportion. Drugs which are unionized can pass through cell membranes to exert their action, while ionized drugs are trapped extracellularly. The acid-base environment and the chemical structure determining whether a drug is acid or base in nature will influence how ionized or unionized a drug is. The pKa is an intrinsic feature of a molecule. It is the pH at which 50% of hydrogen ions are dissociated from the molecule. Acids will exist in the unionized state below their pKa. In contrast, bases will exist in the unionized state above their pKa. Elimination of drugs occurs when the drug is removed from the plasma by the kidneys unchanged or when it is metabolized (usually by the liver).

Further reading

Hardman JG, Hopkins PM, Stuys MMRF. Oxford Textbook of Anaesthesia. Oxford University Press, 2017. Drug distribution and elimination in anaesthetic practice.

Table 2.1 Drug comparison table of the common intravenous induction agents

	pH	pKa	% Unionized at physiological pH	% Protein binding	Volume of distribution L/kg	Half life	Clearance
Propofol	7.4	11.0	99.7	98	4	9.3–69.3 mins	18.8–40.3 ml/kg/min
Ketamine	3.5–5.5	7.5	44	20–50	3	2.5 hours	17 ml/kg/min
Thiopental	10.8	7.6	61	65–86	1.96	3.4–22 hours	2.7–4.1 ml/kg/min
Etomidate	8.1	4.2	99	76.5	4.5	1–4.7 hours	870–1700 ml/min

Smith S, Scarth E. *Drugs in Anaesthesia and Intensive Care*, 5th edition. Oxford University Press, 2016. Etomidate, Ketamine, Propofol, Thiopental.

Williams GW, Williams ES. *Basic Anesthesiological Examination Review*. Oxford University Press, 2015. General concepts in pharmacology.

4. TFTFT

Co-induction is the administration of two or more synergistic classes of drugs in order to induce general anaesthesia. Advantages of this technique include i) benefiting from the effect profile of the separate drugs; ii) reducing the doses of the drugs required to a greater degree than could be achieved with one drug.

Midazolam, if given 90–120 seconds prior to propofol induction, will reduce the amount of propofol required by 30–40%. Opioids and clonidine have been shown to reduce the required amount of propofol for induction and may improve the conditions for siting of supraglottic airways.

Ondansetron has no effect on the administered propofol dose and is non-sedative. Ephedrine, in contrast, has a stimulatory effect that is similar to that of amphetamine.

Further reading

Hardman JG, Hopkins PM, Stuys MMRF. Oxford Textbook of Anaesthesia. Oxford University Press, 2017. Management of anaesthesia.

Smith S, Scarth E. *Drugs in Anaesthesia and Intensive Care*, 5th edition. Oxford University Press, 2016. Ephedrine, Ondansetron, Propofol.

5. TFFFT

Propofol is a phenol derivative. A phenol is a phenyl ring with a hydroxyl group at the first carbon. Propofol has two isopropyl groups at carbons 2 and 6. Propofol preparations contain 100 mg/ml soybean oil, 12 mg/ml egg lecithin, 1 mg benzyl alcohol, 22.5 mg/ml glycerol, and sodium hydroxide to adjust the pH. It is highly lipid soluble with an octanol:water partition coefficient of 6761:1 at a pH of 6–8.

Propofol can only be administered intravenously with a suggested dose for induction of 1–2.5 mg/kg in adults, with a 50% dose increase for children.

Propofol rapidly results in the induction of general anaesthesia with an offset of effects after 10 minutes due to redistribution. Propofol is highly lipid soluble and has a large V_D. It is rapidly metabolized in the liver to inactive glucuronide and sulphate conjugates and quinols via the CYP450 system. It is likely that extrahepatic metabolism occurs. The hepatic extraction ratio is >0.89, and the clearance of propofol is 18.8–40.3 ml/kg/min. Hepatic disease has no significant clinical effect on its metabolism.

Further reading

Hardman JG, Hopkins PM, Stuys MMRF. *Oxford Textbook of Anaesthesia*. Oxford University Press, 2017. Intravenous anaesthetics.

Smith S, Scarth E. *Drugs in Anaesthesia and Intensive Care*, 5th edition, Oxford University Press, 2016. Propofol.

6. TTTFT

Propofol infusion syndrome is a complex of symptoms and signs that develops as a result of propofol infusion. It is not currently clear whether this is because of the propofol itself, or the additives present in the preparation. It typically occurs at day three but with a range of 1–6 days. The annual incidence is estimated as 1.1% with mortality rates of 18%. There is an apparently higher incidence in the paediatric population.

Clinical features include:

- intractable bradycardia
- arrhythmias
- metabolic (usually lactic) acidosis
- rhabdomyolysis
- myoglobinuria
- hyperlipidaemia
- fatty liver
- ECG changes similar to Brugada syndrome (convex ST elevation in V1–3)
- T-wave inversion if circulatory failure develops
- multiorgan failure

The exact aetiology remains unclear, but it is thought to result from impaired mitochondrial fatty acid chain uptake and through an uncoupling of intracellular oxidative phosphorylation and energy production inhibiting electron flow.

Treatment is largely supportive, involving discontinuation of propofol and instituting organ support as required.

Further reading

Loh NHW, Nair P. Propofol infusion syndrome. BJA Education, 2013;13(6):200–202.

Smith S, Scarth E. *Drugs in Anaesthesia and Intensive Care*, 5th edition. Oxford University Press, 2016. Propofol.

7. FTFTT

The physiochemical properties of drugs are determined by the functional groups present in the molecule. This will govern its solubility and stability in solution. Incompatibility is a reversible physiochemical change that occurs due to any of a number of factors including change in pH, dilution of co-solvent, salting out, and cation-anion interactions. This may result in precipitation or insolubility, which may not always be visible, and may occur slowly. It may lead to a reduced effect of the active compound through irreversible chemical degradation.

Ketamine and thiopental are pharmaceutically incompatible and should not be mixed. Mivacurium is incompatible with alkaline solutions and so should not be mixed with thiopental. Rocuronium has several incompatibilities, including thiopental, dexamethasone, erythromycin, vancomycin, and diazepam.

Further reading

Dickman A, Schneider J. *The Syringe Driver: Continuous Subcutaneous Infusions in Palliative Care*, 4th edition. Oxford University Press, 2016. Chemistry of drug incompatibility and stability.

Smith S, Scarth E. Drugs in Anaesthesia *and* Intensive Care, 5th edition. Oxford University Press, 2016. Ketamine, Mivacurium, Rocuronium, Suxamethonium.

Single Best Answers

1. A

Etomidate may produce generalized epileptiform activity on electro-encephalogram (EEG) in 20% of patients. Induction may be associated with involuntary muscle movements in up to 50% of patients, along with tremor and hypertonus. Although up to 10% of patients given propofol may manifest excitatory dystonic movements, EEG does not indicate seizure activity and it is likely that propofol has anticonvulsant properties. Ketamine produces dissociative anaesthesia and patients typically exhibit pupillary dilatation, nystagmus, eyes remaining open, and hypertonus. EEG does not demonstrate seizure activity with its use. Thiopental and midazolam have anticonvulsant effects and do not produce involuntary movements.

Further reading

Smith S, Scarth E. Drugs in Anaesthesia *and* Intensive Care, 5th edition. Oxford University Press, 2016. Etomidate, Ketamine, Propofol, Thiopental.

2. E

Ketamine causes dissociative anaesthesia. It leads to increased cerebral blood flow, metabolic rate, intracranial and intraocular pressure. It typically causes tachycardia and increased vascular tone. Apnoeas are uncommon and it is traditionally said to preserve airway reflexes. There is bronchial smooth muscle relaxation and bronchodilation. Gastric mobility is unchanged while uterine tone is increased. Salivation is a common problem and an antisialagogue may be used prior to administration to reduce this feature. Pain on injection may occur and postoperative nausea and vomiting is common. Movement at induction and hiccups are unlikely to occur. The incidence of hallucinations, restlessness, unpleasant dreams, and emergence delirium may be reduced by premedication with a benzodiazepine.

Further reading

Hardman JG, Hopkins PM, Stuys MMRF. *Oxford Textbook of Anaesthesia*. Oxford University Press, 2017. Intravenous anaesthetics.

Smith S, Scarth E. *Drugs in Anaesthesia and Intensive Care*, 5th edition. Oxford University Press, 2016. Ketamine.

3. **D**

Etomidate is a potent inhibitor of steroid synthesis, both after a bolus or infusion. This is because of inhibition of the enzyme 11-β-hydroxylase which is responsible for cortisol synthesis from 11-deoxycortisol. This effect lasts for 24–48 hours. It is likely that because of this, etomidate has been linked to increased mortality following infusion. However, there is no conclusive evidence to suggest a single dose is linked with morbidity or mortality.

Cortisol is produced in the zona fasiculata of the adrenal gland. All steroid hormone synthesis begins with cholesterol. Initially side chains are cleaved to produce pregnenolone. This is converted to 17-α-hydroxypregnenolone by 17-α-hydroxylase. 3-β-hydroxysteroid dehydrogenase converts this to 17-α-hydroxyprogesterone, which is converted to 11-deoxycortisol by 21-hydroxylase. 11-β-hydroxylase produces cortisol from 11-deoxycortisol.

The adrenal androgens and oestrogens are produced in the zona reticularis. 5-α-reductase produces dihydrotestosterone, while aromatase produces oestradiol and estrone from testosterone and androstenedione.

Further reading

Hardman JG, Hopkins PM, Stuys MMRF. *Oxford Textbook of Anaesthesia*. Oxford University Press, 2017. Intravenous anaesthetics.

Herring N, Wilkins R. *Basic Science for Core Medical Training and the MRCP*. Oxford University Press, 2015. Endocrinology.

Smith S, Scarth E. *Drugs in Anaesthesia and Intensive Care*, 5th edition. Oxford University Press, 2016. Etomidate.

4. **B**

The barbiturate ring structure is formed from malonic acid and urea. Barbiturates can be divided into four main groups based on the side groups of this structure, which confer various properties.

Thiopental is a thiobarbiturate and has a hydrogen at N1 and a sulphur atom at C2. The sulphur group confers increased lipid solubility and so results in increased potency and onset of action. In contrast methohexital, a methylbarbiturate, gains anticonvulsant properties through a methyl side group at N1 and oxygen at C2, while a fatty acid chain leads to greater lipid solubility. Oxybarbiturates have a hydrogen at

N1 and oxygen at C2 and have a slower onset and more prolonged duration of action. Methylthiobarbiturates are not used in clinical practice as they show marked excitatory effects.

Further reading

Gupta A, Singh-Radcliff N. *Pharmacology in Anaesthesia Practice*. Oxford University Press, 2013. Barbiturates.

Hardman JG, Hopkins PM, Stuys MMRF. *Oxford Textbook of Anaesthesia*. Oxford University Press, 2017. Intravenous anaesthetics.

5. A

N-methyl D-aspartate (NMDA) receptors are excitatory ionotropic receptors located within the central nervous system. Glutamate, which is stimulated in response to noxious peripheral stimuli, acts as an agonist at these receptors. Their activation leads to an influx of calcium and cellular depolarization. Ketamine is a non-competitive antagonist of the NMDA receptor calcium channel pore, but also inhibits channel action through a specific receptor binding site. It is independent of glutamate, and so its action cannot be overcome by increased neurotransmitter concentrations. It provides both supraspinal and spinal analgesia and produces dissociative anaesthesia. There is also evidence to suggest that ketamine has several other mechanisms of action, including antagonism at monoaminergic, opioid, muscarinic, and nicotinic receptors. In higher doses it may also act as a sodium channel blocker.

Further reading

Hardman JG, Hopkins PM, Stuys MMRF. *Oxford Textbook of Anaesthesia*. Oxford University Press, 2017. Intravenous anaesthetics.

Ruskin KJ, Rosenbaum SH, Rampil IJ. *Fundamentals of Neuroanaesthesia: A Physiologic Approach to Clinical Practice*. Oxford University Press, 2013. Pharmacology of intravenous sedative-hypnotic agents.

Smith S, Scarth E. *Drugs in Anaesthesia and Intensive Care*, 5th edition. Oxford University Press, 2016. Ketamine.

6. C

Propofol has many desirable features, particularly for neurosurgical patients. Propofol administration results in reduced intracranial pressure (ICP), reduced CMR, and reduced CPP. It does not interfere with cerebral autoregulation. When compared to volatiles, propofol administration results in relatively higher cerebral perfusion pressures with lower ICP and less cerebral oedema.

In contrast, ketamine increases cerebral blood flow and ICP. CMR increases as a result of increased synaptic activation. Despite this, there is no convincing evidence that ketamine is contraindicated in the brain-injured patient for this reason and the cardiovascular stability provided by it is likely to be beneficial.

Etomidate and thiopental decrease ICP, CBF, and CMR for oxygen.

Further reading

Ruskin KJ, Rosenbaum SH, Rampil IJ. *Fundamentals of Neuroanaesthesia: A Physiologic Approach to Clinical Practice*. Oxford University Press, 2013. Pharmacology of intravenous sedative-hypnotic agents.

7. A

Thiopental has a rapid action due to high blood flow to the brain, lipophilicity, and relatively low degree of ionization. The duration is brief and this is mainly due to redistribution to other tissues from the plasma, based on their local blood flow, tissue partition coefficients, and the blood-tissue gradients. Thiopental is hepatically metabolized by side-arm oxidation, oxidation to pentobarbital, and ring cleavage to form urea and 3-carbon fragments via the CYP450 system.

It is not suitable for TIVA due to its low hepatic extraction ratio. Thiopental clearance is dependent on hepatic clearance (roughly 15% being metabolized per hour) rather than hepatic blood flow. At high concentrations clearance assumes zero-order kinetics due to enzyme saturation. This combined with its relatively high V_D result in accumulation of the drug and therefore very slow offset with infusion or repeated doses.

Further reading

Hardman JG, Hopkins PM, Stuys MMRF. *Oxford Textbook of Anaesthesia*. Oxford University Press, 2017. Intravenous anaesthetics.

Smith S, Scarth E. *Drugs in Anaesthesia and Intensive Care*, 5th edition, Oxford University Press, 2016. Thiopental.

Local anaesthetic agents

QUESTIONS

Multiple-Choice Questions

1. The following statements about ropivacaine are true:

A Ropivacaine is available as racemic and enantio-pure preparations

B The pKa of ropivacaine is 9.4

C The recommended maximal dose is 2 mg/kg

D The addition of sodium bicarbonate to ropivacaine will significantly increase its duration of action

E The combination of adrenaline with ropivacaine increases the maximal recommended dose threshold

2. Local anaesthetics have been associated with the following effects:

A Antithrombosis

B Anti-inflammatory action

C Prevention of lung injury

D Antimicrobial effects

E Reduced airway hyper-responsiveness in asthmatics

3. Regarding 2-chloroprocaine

A Is an amide anaesthetic

B Duration of action is similar to low-dose bupivacaine for spinal anaesthesia

C In common with cocaine, it has vasoconstrictor actions

D Should be avoided in patients taking trimethoprim

E Serum half-life is prolonged with co-administration of IV morphine

4. The following statements relating to local anaesthetic toxicity are correct:

A The S-enantiomer of bupivacaine binds with less affinity to cardiac sodium channels than the R+ enantiomer

B Risk of toxicity is influenced by the site of injection where intercostal > epidural > caudal > brachial plexus

C Doses of local anaesthetics should be reduced by 15% for patients aged <4 months old

D Administration of 18 ml 2% lidocaine + 1:200,000 adrenaline would be considered within recommended maximal dose parameters for a 60 kg adult

E The cardiovascular collapse: seizure dose ratio (CC:CNS) is 7.1:1 for lidocaine

5. Regarding local anaesthetics

A The ionized form of local anaesthetic has a high affinity for resting-state sodium channels

B The membrane expansion theory is mediated by the unionized drug fraction

C A-alpha nerve fibres are less susceptible to blockade by local anaesthetics than A-delta fibres

D Procaine is an agonist at the N-methyl D-aspartate (NMDA) receptor

E Local anaesthetic agents have been shown to inhibit the ryanodine receptor at the sarcoplasmic reticulum

6. The following statements about lidocaine are true

A Fluconazole reduces plasma clearance of lidocaine

B Is effectively removed by haemodialysis

C Is more likely to trigger an allergic reaction than benzocaine

D Cimetidine can increase the blood concentration of lidocaine

E Is safe to use in patients with porphyria

7. Regarding the use of cocaine as a local anaesthetic:

A Cocaine is hydrolysed by serum and hepatic esterases

B In common with many local anaesthetics, cocaine has a biphasic vasoactive effect

C The toxic dose is 3 mg/kg for topical administration

D Is antiemetic

E Increases body temperature through direct actions on the pons

Single Best Answers

1. Which of the following is the best definition for pKa?

A The acid dissociation constant

B The negative logarithm of the base dissociation constant of an alkaline solution

C The pH at which 50% of molecules exist in the ionized form and 50% exist in the unionized form

D The pH at which the drug is 100% associated with an acidic compound

E The pH at which the drug undergoes autoionization

2. A 55-year-old patient presents to the emergency department six hours following a day case operation. She is complaining of a headache, fatigue, and mild dyspnoea. Her oxygen saturation at room air record at 85%. An arterial blood gas is noted to look 'chocolate' in colour when it is taken and returns a value of 14.8 kPa PO_2.

Which of the following drugs do you consider most likely that the patient has been given, which could account for her presentation?

A 2-chlorprocaine

B EMLA™ cream

C Prilocaine

D Proxymetacaine

E Ropivacaine

3. Which of the following statements about the physicochemical properties of local anaesthetics is the most accurate?

A Aliphatic substitutions in the aromatic ring enhance potency

B Increasing hydrocarbon chain length reduces lipid solubility

C Protein binding primarily determines the speed of onset

D The potency of a local anaesthetic is primarily determined by its pKa value

E The addition of sodium bicarbonate to an amide local anaesthetic increases the ionized fraction

4. A patient complains of perioral tingling and auditory disturbance approx. four mins after an interscalene nerve block has been performed. She rapidly loses consciousness, convulses, and broad complexes are noted on her electrocardiograph (ECG). Treatment for local anaesthetic systemic toxicity is instituted. The patient weighs 60 kg.

Which of the following is the most appropriate initial treatment regimen?

A 10% lipid emulsion: 60 ml IV bolus + infusion of 600 ml/hr

B 10% lipid emulsion: 100 ml IV bolus + infusion of 1000 ml/hr

C 20% lipid emulsion: 90 ml IV bolus + infusion of 900 ml/hr

D 20% lipid emulsion: 90 ml IV bolus + infusion of 1800 ml/hr

E 20% lipid emulsion: 120 ml IV bolus, repeated at 5 min intervals for a further two doses

5. A 28-year-old male has an area of inflamed, acidotic tissue, which requires a local anaesthetic to allow the removal of a foreign body. Which local anaesthetic drug is most likely to be effective?

A Amethocaine

B Levobupivacaine

C Lidocaine

D Mepivacaine

E Procaine

6. Concerning binding plasma binding of local anaesthetics, which of the following statements is the most accurate statement?

A Albumin binds local anaesthetics with higher affinity than α_1-acid glycoprotein

B Foetal ion trapping is more likely with bupivacaine than lidocaine

C Higher unbound fractions of local anaesthetics would be expected in pregnancy

D Neonates have approximately 25% of the adult plasma concentration of α_1-acid glycoprotein

E Patients with severe renal impairment have a reduced concentration of α_1-acid glycoprotein

7. You are told that a local anaesthetic agent 'Y' has a percentage unionized fraction at pH 7.4 of 25%. Which of the following pKa values is this agent 'Y' most likely to have?

A pKa = 7.6

B pKa = 7.9

C pKa = 8.1

D pKa = 8.7

E pKa = 8.9

ANSWERS

Multiple-Choice Questions

1. TFFTF

Ropivacaine has a pKa of 8.1, a maximal recommended dose of 3 mg/ kg and is available as racemic and an 'S' enantiopure preparation (the S-isomer is less cardiotoxic and more potent than the 'R' isomer). Alkalinization of ropivacaine increases its duration of action. The addition of adrenaline however does not increase the recommended dose threshold or the duration of effect. Ropivacaine has intrinsic vasoconstrictive properties.

Further reading

Smith S, Scarth E. *Drugs in Anaesthesia and Intensive Care*, 5th edition. Oxford University Press, 2016. Ropivacaine.

2. TTTTT

Local anaesthetics have been associated with antithrombotic actions, including reduced platelet aggregation and reduced maximum amplitude recordings on thromboelastography. They have also been shown to reduce inflammation via non-sodium channel-mediated mechanisms. Leucocyte adhesion and migration, cell signalling with protein kinase C/phospholipase D, and phagocytosis have all been shown to reduce with local anaesthetics. Prevention of acute lung injury and myocardial injury has also been shown with local anaesthetic agents. Bacterial inhibition of various strains of pathogens has also been demonstrated (e.g. *Pseudomonas*, *E.coli*, and *Staph aureus*) as have antiviral and antifungal effects. The mechanism of reduced airway hyper-responsiveness is thought to be the vagal blockade of bronchoconstriction reflexes.

Further reading

Cassuto J, Sinclair R, Bonderovic M. Anti-inflammatory properties of local anesthetics and their present and potential clinical implications. *Acta Anaesthesiol Scand*, 2006;50:265–282.

Hollmann MW, Durieux ME. Local anesthetics and the inflammatory response: a new therapeutic indication? *Anesthesiology*, 2000;93:858–875.

3. FFFTT

2-chloroprocaine is an ester local anaesthetic agent. It has a rapid onset time and a short duration of action. It is commonly used as a spinal anaesthetic agent to facilitate day-case surgery. The typical time to onset is 3–5 minutes, motor block duration of 40 minutes, and time to ambulation 90 minutes. When compared with low-dose spinal bupivacaine, 2-chloroprocaine has a similar onset time but a faster offset time. Cocaine is a vasoconstrictor, however chloroprocaine is a vasodilator. The para-aminobenzoic acid metabolite of chloroprocaine inhibits the action of sulfonamides and may decrease their therapeutic effect. Examples of drugs in this class include trimethoprim, sulfonylureas, some diuretics (e.g. bumetanide) and antiretrovirals. Morphine has been found to inhibit pseudocholinesterase by up to 5%. Pseudocholinesterase hydrolyses the ester linkage in 2-chloroprocaine and thus any inhibition of pseudo-cholinesterase will prolong the serum half-life of 2-chloroprocaine. This has not clinically been shown to be of significance.

Further reading

Bailey D, Briggs JR. Studies of the inhibition of serum pseudocholin-esterase activity in vitro by commonly used drugs. *Am J Clin Pathol*, 2005;124:226–228.

Smith S, Scarth E. *Drugs in Anaesthesia and Intensive Care*, 5th edition. Oxford University Press, 2016. Chloroprocaine.

4. TFTTT

Levobupivacaine comprises only the S-enantiomer and has been mar-keted as an enantiopure preparation due to its enhanced cardiac safety benefits. The risk of toxicity reactions is influenced by the block site; however, the correct 'risk order' is intercostal > caudal > epidural > brachial plexus. Neonates and infants <4 months old should have doses of local anaesthetic reduced by 15% due to immature hepatic enzyme systems and reduced plasma protein binding.

Maximal recommended doses are 3 mg/kg for lidocaine without adren-aline and 7 mg/kg for lidocaine + adrenaline. While the lowest possible dose should always be used, this patient's maximal dose would be 420 mg, therefore the 360 mg dose presented is within acceptable limits. The CC:CNS dose ratio shows the differences in the dose required to produce cardiovascular collapse vs. induce seizures. For lidocaine, this is quoted as 7.1. Bupivacaine is much more likely to progress from central nervous system signs to cardiovascular collapse as shown by its CC:CNS ratio of just 2.

Further reading

Christie LE, Picard J, Weinberg GL. Local anaesthetic systemic toxicity. Cont Educ Anaesth Crit Care *Pain*, 2015;15(3):136–142.

El-Boghdadly K, Pawa A, Chin KJ. Local anesthetic systemic toxicity: cur-rent perspectives. *Local Reg Anesth*, 2018;11:35–44.

Smith S, Scarth E. *Drugs in Anaesthesia and Intensive Care*, 5th edition. Oxford University Press, 2016. Lidocaine.

5. FTTFT

Sodium channels may be in the open, inactive, or resting state. Local anaesthetic agents have the greatest affinity for sodium channels in their open or inactive states. Blockade occurs from within the cell—the unionized form of the local anaesthetic drug diffuses into the cell. There it becomes protonated (ionized) and blocks the sodium channel thus preventing action potential conduction. Nerve fibres with high rates of firing are more likely to have sodium channels in the non-resting state and thus be susceptible to local anaesthetic blockade (e.g. pain fibres, cardiac pacemaker cells). Equally cells with long action potentials are more likely to have 'open' sodium channels (again seen in pain fibres and cardiac muscle cells). A-alpha fibres are large-diameter nerve fibres and also have much shorter action potential durations. For both of these reasons, they are much less likely to be blocked by local anaesthetic agents than the smaller long-action potential a-delta fibres.

It is the unionized drug fraction which is thought to interact with the cell membrane from outside of the cell (membrane expansion theory) and also disrupt action potential conduction. Procaine is an antagonist at NMDA receptors. Local anaesthetic agents have indeed been shown to modulate the ryanodine receptor and reduce calcium-dependent myofilament contractility. Other demonstrated effects include inhibition of mitochondrial metabolism and various cell signalling mechanisms.

Further reading

El-Boghdadly K, Pawa A, Chin KJ. Local anesthetic systemic toxicity: current perspectives. *Local Reg Anesth*, 2018;11:35–44.

6. TFFTT

Amide local anaesthetics are hepatically metabolized by the cytochrome p450 system. Fluconazole inhibits CYP3A4 hence co-administration will reduce lidocaine plasma clearance by up to 15% although this is rarely clinically of significance. Lidocaine is not removed by haemodialysis. True IgE-mediated local anaesthetic allergy to amides is very rare (<1% all reported reactions). Ester anaesthetics (e.g. benzocaine) are more likely to produce allergic reactions as they are metabolized to para-amino benzoic acid (PABA) which is highly antigenic. PABA is also found in many cosmetics/toiletries products and may immunologically presensitize individuals. Preservatives in amide anaesthetics, e.g. sodium metabisulphite, methylparaben, have also been implicated in reactions.

Cimetidine inhibits CYP 2D6 which can lead to reduced amide metabolism and raised blood levels. Porphyria is a rare hereditary disorder of haem synthesis. Porphyric crises can be triggered by a number of drugs; however, lidocaine is on the 'safe' drugs list for this condition.

Further reading

Bhole MV, Manson AL, Seneviratne SL, Misbah SA. IgE-mediated allergy to local anaesthetics: separating fact from perception: a UK perspective. *Br J Anaesth*, 2012;108(6):903–911.

Drugs in Porphyria. Available at: https://www.wmic.wales.nhs.uk/specialist-services/drugs-in-porphyria/

Smith S, Scarth E, Sasada S. *Drugs in Anaesthesia and Intensive Care*, 5th edition. Oxford University Press, 2016. Lidocaine.

7. TFTFF

Cocaine blocks sodium channels to function as a local anaesthetic; it also inhibits noradrenaline, serotonin, and dopamine reuptake. Esters local anaesthetics are generally metabolized exclusively in the plasma, however, cocaine differs as it is hydrolysed by both serum and hepatic esterases. Also, in contrast to the typically biphasic vasoactive profile of local anaesthetics (i.e. at low doses they are vasoconstrictive to peripheral vascular smooth muscle and at higher doses vasodilatory), cocaine is purely vasoconstrictive. Use is associated with nausea, abdominal pain, and gastrointestinal upset—this is thought to be part centrally mediated and part gut ischaemia from its vasoconstrictive actions. Hyperthermia is commonly associated due to both cutaneous vasoconstriction and direct action at the hypothalamus.

Further reading

Smith S, Scarth E. *Drugs in Anaesthesia and Intensive Care*, 5th edition. Oxford University Press, 2016. Cocaine.

Single Best Answers

1. C

pKa is the negative log of the acid dissociation constant Ka. So A would be the correct definition of Ka but not pKa. Autoionization is a process where electrons are spontaneously emitted from an outer electron shell when an atom or molecule is in an excited state and thus changes its charge from a neutral to an ionized ($^{+1}$) state.

Further reading

Taylor A, McLeod G. Basic pharmacology of local anaesthetics. *BJA Education*, 2020;20(2):34–41.

2. C

The diagnosis here is methaemoglobinaemia and the most likely causative agent from the list given here is prilocaine. Other causative drug agents include: benzocaine, lidocaine, tetracaine, phenytoin, metoclopramide, sulphonamides, sodium nitroprusside, and glyceryl trinitrate.

Prilocaine generates O-toluidine which oxidizes Hb. Peak levels of MetHb occur approximately 4–8 hours following administration. EMLA™ cream is also a recognized trigger (as it contains prilocaine) but given the mass of an adult and the likely maximum amount of EMLA™ that could have been applied, prilocaine is a much more likely option.

Methaemoglobinaemia is a condition where the Fe^{2+} ions of haem are oxidized from ferrous to ferric Fe^{3+}. This renders them unable to bind oxygen, left shifts the oxy-haemoglobin dissociation curve, and makes it more difficult for oxygen to be released to tissues. Low levels of methaemoglobin (MetHb) are normal (<1%) but levels >40% can become life-threatening.

Significant methaemoglobinaemia is more common in infants, with co-administration of other causative agents, repeated doses, and in pre-existing anaemia/haemoglobinopathies. Management is treatment with methylene blue. This provides an artificial electron transporter which reduces MetHb to Hb. The dose is 1–2 mg/kg IV. Methylthioninium chloride is contraindicated in patients with glucose-6-phosphate dehydrogenase (G6PD) deficiency. Other treatments induce hyperbaric oxygen and exchange transfusion.

Further reading

Alanazi MQ. Drugs may be induced methaemoglobinaemia. *J Hematol Thrombo Dis*, 2017;5:3.

Smith S, Scarth E. *Drugs in Anaesthesia and Intensive Care*, 5th edition. Oxford University Press, 2016. Prilocaine.

3. A

An agent's pKa determines the percentage of drug which will be unionized at physiological pH and thus primarily influences the speed of onset. Protein binding influences the duration of action with highly protein-bound drugs tending to have longer durations of action. Alkalinization will environmentally create a pH closer to the agent's pKa and therefore proportionally increases the unionized drug fraction. Increasing hydrocarbon chain length and aromatic ring aliphatic substitutions will increase lipid solubility. Lipid solubility is primarily associated with a local anaesthetic agent's potency.

Further reading

Taylor A, McLeod G. Basic pharmacology of local anaesthetics. *BJA Education*, 2020;20(2):34–41.

4. C

AAGBI guidelines recommend treatment with 20% lipid emulsion IV. The regimen is 1.5 ml/kg as an IV bolus over 1 minute, followed by an infusion of 15 ml/kg/hr. After 5 minutes further boluses doses may be repeated (×2 more = total of three doses) and the infusion rate doubled to 30 ml/kg/hr. Maximal doses of 12 ml/kg are not recommended to be exceeded. Other supportive care including airway management +/− prolonged cardiopulmonary resuscitation may also be required.

Further reading

AAGBI Management of Severe Local Aanesthetic Toxicity Guidelines, 2010. Available at: https://www.aagbi.org/sites/default/files/la_toxicity_2010_0.pdf

Smith S, Scarth E. *Drugs in Anaesthesia and Intensive Care*, 5th edition. Oxford University Press, 2016. Intralipid® 20%.

5. D

All local anaesthetic drugs have a pKa greater than 7.4, meaning more than 50% exist in the water soluble ionized form. In an acidic environment, even fewer drug molecules will exist in the lipid-soluble unionized form. Thus the drug with the lowest pKa will be the most effective as it will proportionally have the most drug molecules in the unionized state. The pKas of the drugs presented are: amethocaine 8.5; levobupivacaine 8.1; lidocaine 7.9; mepivacaine 7.6; and procaine 8.9. Therefore, mepivacaine is most likely to be effective.

Further reading

Smith S, Scarth E. *Drugs in Anaesthesia and Intensive Care*, 5th edition. Oxford University Press, 2016. APPENDIX A1.3.

6. C

Plasma binding of local anaesthetic agents reduces the free fraction and hence the risk of toxicity reactions occurring. α_1-acid glycoprotein has a higher affinity for binding local anaesthetics, but albumin binds a greater fraction due to its abundance. Neonates have approximately 50% of the adult level of α_1-acid glycoprotein which means they have an increased risk of toxicity and delayed elimination. Pregnancy reduces levels of albumin and α_1-acid glycoprotein which increases the unbound fraction of local anaesthetics. Patients with severe renal impairment actually have elevated levels of α_1-acid glycoprotein, although remain at increased risk of toxicity reactions due to reduced renal clearance. Placental transfer of lidocaine is greater than for bupivacaine as there is a higher free fraction of drug (lower maternal protein binding of lidocaine) and a higher % unionized fraction at maternal pH 7.4 due to the lower pKa of lidocaine, thus risk of an acidotic foetus trapping ions is lower with bupivacaine.

Further reading

Christie LE, Picard J, Weinberg GL. Local anaesthetic systemic toxicity. *Cont Educ Anaesth Crit Care Pain*, 2015;15(3):136–142.

Johnson RF, et al. Effects of fetal pH on local anaesthetic transfer across the human placenta. *Anaesthesiology*, 1996;85:608–615.

Smith S, Scarth E. *Drugs in Anaesthesia and Intensive Care*, 5th edition. Oxford University Press, 2016. APPENDIX A1.3.

7. B

The pKa describes the pH at which 50% of the drug molecules exist in the ionized form and 50% exist in the unionized form. All local anaesthetic drugs are weak bases with pKa values greater than 7.4. The closer the agent's pKa value is to pH 7.4 the closer to 50% unionized the drug fraction will be. Drugs with a high pKa will have a much smaller percentage of drug unionized at physiological pH 7.4. The drug being described is actually lidocaine, which at pH 7.4 is 25% unionized but at pH 7.0 would be ~11% unionized.

For comparison: mepivacaine (pKa 7.6) is 39% unionized at pH 7.4, bupivacaine (pKa 8.1) is 15% unionized, and chloroprocaine (pKa 8.7) is 4.8% unionized.

Further reading

Smith S, Scarth E. *Drugs in Anaesthesia and Intensive Care*, 5th edition. Oxford University Press, 2016. Lidocaine.

Werdehausen R, et al. Apoptosis induction by different local anaesthetics in a neuroblastoma cell line. *Br J Anaesth*, 2009;103(5):711–718.

Drugs affecting neuromuscular function

QUESTIONS

Multiple-Choice Questions

1. For sugammadex:

A A dose of 4 mg/kg is recommended when recovery of neuromuscular function has reached T2

B The recommended dose for 'rescue reversal' in a 'can't intubate, can't oxygenate' scenario is 16 mg/kg

C Dose calculation should be based on ideal body weight

D A dose reduction is recommended in older people

E Less than 30% of a given dose is excreted within 24 hours

2. Rocuronium

A Is a benzylisoquinolinium

B Is less potent than atracurium

C Dose calculation should be based on ideal body weight in morbidly obese patients

D Has a higher volume of distribution compared to atracurium

E Pain on injection with rocuronium is worse in conjunction with propofol compared to thiopental

3. Regarding the effective dosages (ED) of neuromuscular blocking agents:

A Double the ED90 dosage of rocuronium should be administered during rapid sequence induction

B ED90 is a measure of drug efficacy

C Rocuronium has an ED90 of 0.3 mg/kg

D The ED90 of rocuronium is greater than that of atracurium

E Standard intubating dose of vecuronium is 0.1 mg/kg

4. Regarding dantrolene:

A The treatment dose for acute malignant hyperthermia is 16 mg/kg

B Is available as a solution containing 2.5 mg/ml

C Inhibits calcium release via the inhibition of ryanodine receptors

D Impairs skeletal muscle action potential

E Mean duration of action is 15 minutes

5. Regarding the metabolism of drugs affecting neuromuscular function:

A Rocuronium has no active metabolites

B Vecuronium is deacetylated in the liver to active metabolites

C The majority of mivacurium isomers are hydrolysed by plasma cholinesterase

D Hofmann degradation is the minor pathway of cisatracurium metabolism

E 30% of suxamethonium is hydrolysed before reaching the neuromuscular junction

6. Neostigmine

A Binds to the anionic site of acetylcholinesterase

B Prolongs the duration of action of suxamethonium

C Peak action occurs within 1–2 minutes post intravenous bolus

D Predominantly undergoes plasma esterase metabolism

E Does not cross the blood–brain barrier

7. Suxamethonium

A Is an ester of succinic acid

B Prevents skeletal muscle action potential repolarization

C Increases lower oesophageal tone

D Is appropriate in the immediate management of a patient with severe burns

E Has a shortened duration of action in pregnancy

Single Best Answers

1. You have performed a modified rapid sequence induction (RSI) of anaesthesia for a 67-year-old patient undergoing rigid oesophagoscopy for a retained food bolus. The procedure proceeds uneventfully and is over within 5 minutes. Which property of rocuronium best informs the 'reversal' dose of sugammadex?

A It is non-cumulative with repeated administration

B Its ED90 is 0.3 mg/kg

C Its effect is augmented by the recent co-administration of propofol

D Rocuronium non-competitively antagonizes acetylcholine at nicotinic (N_2) receptors

E The recovery index of an RSI dose reaches 1 hour

2. You have anaesthetised a 24-year-old woman for a laparoscopic cholecystectomy. Following completion of the procedure you conduct a quantitative train-of-four analysis. This elicits two twitches. Regarding the reversal of neuromuscular antagonism due to rocuronium, which of the following statements represents optimal management?

A Administer glycopyrronium 500 mcg/neostigmine 0.05–0.07 mg/kg

B Administer sugammadex 2 mg/kg

C Administer sugammadex 4 mg/kg

D Administer sugammadex 16 mg/kg

E Delay administration of glycopyrronium 500 mcg/neostigmine 0.05–0.07 mg/kg

3. Which of the following features best characterizes a suxamethonium-induced phase I neuromuscular block?

A Poorly sustained tetanus during stimulation

B Reversibility with anticholinesterases

C Tachyphylaxis

D The absence of post-tetanic facilitation

E Train-of-four ratio of <0.3

4. A 32-year-old female is undergoing a laparoscopic appendicectomy on the emergency list. She was given suxamethonium as part of her anaesthetic induction. Two hours later at the end of surgery, you try to wake the patient. Her observations are pulse 120, BP 165/95, but no return of spontaneous ventilation. What is the most likely explanation?

A The effect of suxamethonium is prolonged as the patient is on the oral contraceptive pill

B The patient has a genotype of Ea:Ea

C The patient has a genotype of Es:Es

D The patient has a genotype of Eu:Ea

E The patient has reduced plasma cholinesterase due to liver disease

5. You are pre-assessing a 68-year-old patient who has severe chronic renal failure. When considering the use of neuromuscular blocking drugs in planning his anaesthetic, which statement is the most accurate?

A Atracurium: elimination half-life will be little altered by renal impairment

B Mivacurium: duration of action increases threefold in renal impairment

C Rocuronium: the mean duration of action will be prolonged with significant renal impairment

D Suxamethonium: 60% will be excreted unchanged in the urine

E Vecuronium: half-life will be unchanged by renal failure

6. A 36-year-old male remains in intensive care six days postoperatively following an emergency fasciotomy to treat compartment syndrome of his right leg caused by a crush injury. He has a background of epilepsy. He remains sedated, facilitating treatment for rhabdomyolysis. His trachea is intubated and ventilated. He has developed acute respiratory distress syndrome (ARDS), for which he is receiving continuous neuromuscular blockade. He is persistently tachycardic at 130 bpm and pyrexic at 39.3°C. His transaminases are elevated and he has developed an acute kidney injury necessitating haemofiltration. Which of the following is best included in the reasoning for administering a cisatracurium infusion to this patient?

A It is safe to administer to those susceptible to malignant hyperthermia

B Its dose does not require alteration in patients with hepatic impairment

C Its duration of action is shortened with chronic anticonvulsant therapy

D Laudanosine levels are lower compared to atracurium

E Levels are minimally altered following haemofiltration

7. You are reviewing a 55-year-old woman in the general medical ward who has been admitted with profound muscle weakness. Edrophonium is considered in facilitating diagnosis. What feature best informs its role in the 'Tensilon® test' in comparison to neostigmine?

A Edrophonium has a more rapid onset of action

B It has reduced potency than neostigmine

C It is hydrolysed by acetylcholinesterase

D It resolves weakness in a cholinergic crisis

E It reversibly binds to acetylcholinesterase

ANSWERS

Multiple-Choice Questions

1. FTFFF

2 mg/kg is recommended when recovery of neuromuscular function has reached T2 (second evoked response on a train-of-four pattern of nerve stimulation). 16 mg/kg is recommended for immediate emergent reversal. In contrast to rocuronium, sugammadex dosing is based on actual body weight. No dose reduction is recommended in elderly patients. The time of recovery of 0.9 T4:T1 ratio may be slightly prolonged. Sugammadex is not recommended for severe renal or hepatic impairment. More than 90% of a given dose is excreted within 24 hours. A 24-hour delay is recommended before repeat dosing of rocuronium.

Further reading

Smith S, Scarth E. *Drugs in Anaesthesia and Intensive Care*, 5th edition. Oxford University Press, 2016. Sugammadex.

2. FTTTT

Rocuronium is an aminosteroid, which is structurally related to vecuronium. Atracurium is a benzylisoquinolinium ester. Rocuronium (ED90 0.3 mg/kg) is less potent than atracurium (ED90 0.19 mg/kg). This fact necessitates the administration of an increased dose. The concentration gradient at the neuromuscular junction is therefore increased, leading to faster diffusion of drug molecules and a reduction in drug onset time. Dose calculation should be based on ideal body weight in morbidly obese patients.

The volume of distribution of rocuronium is 0.27 L/kg, while that of atracurium is 0.16–0.18 L/kg. 16% of patients experience pain on injection of rocuronium in combination with propofol, compared to 0.5% of patients when used in conjunction with thiopental.

Further reading

Smith S, Scarth E. *Drugs in Anaesthesia and Intensive Care*, 5th edition. Oxford University Press, 2016. Rocuronium.

3. FFTFT

Rocuronium has an ED90 of 0.3 mg/kg. Doubling the ED90 dose is recommended for non-emergent induction of anaesthesia. This results in excellent intubating conditions within 60 seconds of administration of rocuronium in 80% of patients. In a modified RSI a dose of 1 mg/kg is recommended, which achieves excellent intubating conditions in 93–96% of cases within 60 seconds.

ED90 is a measure of drug potency. It is the dose of drug required to produce a 90% reduction in twitch height, whereas efficacy describes the maximal response attainable from a given drug.

Atracurium has an ED90 of 0.19 mg/kg, significantly less than the ED90 of rocuronium, thus rocuronium is a less potent drug than atracurium. The ED90 of vecuronium is 0.057 mg/kg. The standard intubating dose of vecuronium is 0.1 mg/kg.

Further reading

Smith S, Scarth E. *Drugs in Anaesthesia and Intensive Care*, 5th edition. Oxford University Press, 2011. Atracurium, Rocuronium, Vecuronium.

4. FFTFF

The treatment dose range of dantrolene is 1–10 mg/kg. 2.5 mg/kg is the average requirement. It is prepared from a lyophilized orange powder (containing 20 mg of dantrolene, 3 g of mannitol, and NaOH), reconstituted with 60 ml of water. Dantrolene acts within skeletal muscle fibres. It inhibits sarcoplasmic reticulum Ca^{2+} release through the inhibition of ryanodine receptors, thereby diminishing the degree of muscular contraction to a given electrical stimulus. It has no effect on the neuronal action potential. It only diminishes the force of electrically induced muscle twitches. Therapeutic benefit is evident within 15 minutes. Its mean duration of action is 4–6 hours.

Further reading

Smith S, Scarth E. *Drugs in Anaesthesia and Intensive Care*, 5th edition. Oxford University Press, 2016. Dantrolene.

5. TTTFF

No active metabolites of rocuronium have been detected in the plasma or urine.

Vecuronium is deacetylated in the liver into active metabolites. 3-hydroxyvecuronium has 50% potency of vecuronium. However, this is present at a minimal concentration, unlikely to have any clinical significance in the absence of prolonged dosing.

Cis-trans and Trans-trans mivacurium isomers are hydrolysed by plasma cholinesterase; the cis-cis isomer is independent of this pathway. Non-specific plasma esterases are also involved in its hydrolysis.

As with atracurium, Hofmann degradation to laudanosine and a quaternary monoacrylate is the major metabolic pathway of cisatracurium.

80% of suxamethonium is hydrolysed before reaching the neuromuscular junction.

Further reading

Smith S, Scarth E. *Drugs in Anaesthesia and Intensive Care*, 5th edition. Oxford University Press, 2016. Cisatracurium, Mivacurium, Rocuronium, Suxamethonium, Vecuronium.

6. FTFTT

Acetylcholinesterases have two types of active site: a peripheral anionic site and a central esteratic site. Neostigmine binds to the esteratic site. Through inhibition of cholinesterase activity, neostigmine potentiates the effects of depolarizing muscle relaxants. Peak action occurs within 7–11 minutes post intravenous bolus. It predominantly undergoes plasma esterase metabolism. A degree of hepatic metabolism and biliary excretion may occur. Neostigmine is highly ionized and therefore does not cross the blood–brain barrier. It has a low volume of distribution (0.4–1 L/kg).

Further reading

Nair VP, Hunter JM. Anticholinesterases and anticholinergic drugs. *Cont Educ Anaesth Crit Care Pain*, 2004;4:164–168.

Smith S, Scarth E. *Drugs in Anaesthesia and Intensive Care*, 5th edition. Oxford University Press, 2016. Neostigmine.

7. TTFTF

Suxamethonium is a dicholine ester of succinic acid. It is the equivalent of two acetylcholine molecules bonded. It causes prolonged depolarization of skeletal muscle fibres to a membrane potential above which an action potential can be triggered. It prevents repolarization and renders the skeletal muscle cell refractory to further depolarization.

It increases intragastric pressure by 7–12 cmH_2O while simultaneously decreasing lower oesophageal tone.

Suxamethonium is safe within the first 24 hours after a burn, after which time a marked hyperkalaemic response may occur. This is thought to be related to increased levels of extrajunctional acetylcholine receptors, which may persist for up to 1 year after a burn.

Plasma cholinesterase hydrolyses suxamethonium. Its concentrations may be reduced in pregnancy, thereby prolonging the action of suxamethonium. Plasma cholinesterase concentrations may also be reduced by genetic factors and in acquired states, such as liver disease, and cardiac or renal failure.

Further reading

Bishop S, Maguire S. Anaesthesia and intensive care for major burns. *Cont Educ Anaesth Crit Care Pain*, 2012;12(3):118–122.

Smith S, Scarth E. *Drugs in Anaesthesia and Intensive Care*, 5th edition. Oxford University Press, 2016. Suxamethonium.

Single Best Answers

1. E

Rocuronium is non-cumulative with repeated administration. This is of little relevance in a case where only one dose would have been required. Its effect is enhanced by the co-administration of various drugs, including volatile anaesthetics, induction agents, fentanyl, and suxamethonium. Although its ED90 is 0.3 mg/kg, this plays an indirect role in necessitating the administration of an increased dose to facilitate RSI. The standard induction dose is 0.6 mg/kg, while that for RSI is 1.2 mg/kg.

The usual recovery index is 8 to 17 minutes following a standard bolus dose. Following 1 mg/kg bolus dose, the recovery index approaches 1 hour.

Rocuronium competitively antagonizes acetylcholine at nicotinic (N_2) receptors at the post-synaptic membrane of the neuromuscular junction. This property facilitates its reversal.

Further reading

Smith S, Scarth E. *Drugs in Anaesthesia and Intensive Care*, 5th edition. Oxford University Press, 2011. Rocuronium.

2. A

Sugammadex decreases the amount of free drug in the central compartment, creating a concentration gradient away from the neuromuscular junction (NMJ) effector site. It is typically utilized to antagonize profound neuromuscular blockade, which would be refractory to neostigmine.

Neostigmine binds to the esteratic site of acetylcholinesterase, allowing accumulation of acetylcholine, thereby antagonizing the effects of non-depolarizing neuromuscular blocking agents, while potentiating the effects of depolarizing agents. Given that two twitches are evident on quantitative train-of-four (TOF) analysis, this suggests there is already sufficient competitive antagonism of neuromuscular blockade occurring that would benefit from the administration of a standard dose combination of glycopyrronium 500 mcg/neostigmine 0.05–0.07 mg/kg. The recommended dose of sugammadex is defined by the clinical context and the number of twitches present on TOF analysis. 16 mg/kg would be the dose required to immediately reverse deep neuromuscular block, for example, in the context of a failed intubation in an RSI using up to 1.2 mg/kg rocuronium.

Further reading

Moi D. Residual Neuromuscular Blockade: Anaesthesia Tutorial of the Week, 2013. Available at: https://www.frca.co.uk/Documents/290%20Residual%20Neuromuscular%20Blockade.pdf

Schaller SJ, Fink H. Sugammadex as a reversal agent for neuromuscular block: an evidence-based review. *Core Evidence*, 2013;8:57–67.

3. D

Suxamethonium induces skeletal muscle fasciculations followed by a phase I depolarizing blockade. This is characterized by well-sustained tetanus during a 50–100 MHz stimulation, with an absence of post-tetanic facilitation. TOF T4/T1 ratio remains greater than 0.7, indicating a lack of fade, in contrast to non-depolarizing neuromuscular blockade. Tachyphylaxis, describing a diminished response to repeated doses, occurs in a phase II block. A phase I block is potentiated by anticholinesterase activity.

Further reading

Smith S, Scarth E. *Drugs in Anaesthesia and Intensive Care*, 5th edition. Oxford University Press, 2016. Suxamethonium.

4. B

The observations indicate she remains paralysed but her elevated pulse rate and blood pressure show that she is developing awareness. Supportive respiratory treatment along with reassurance to the patient and re-anaesthesia is required. The most likely explanation is that she has a genetic variant of plasma cholinesterase and has a prolonged response to suxamethonium. Genetic testing of the patient and their family should be subsequently offered.

There are four alleles, the inheritance pattern of which produces 10 genotypes. 94-96% of the white population is homozygous Eu:Eu and rapidly metabolizes suxamethonium in <8 mins. The other three alleles are Ea (atypical), Es (silent) and Ef (fluoride resistant). Eu:Ea has a population incidence of 1:25 but seldom prolongs suxamethonium effect beyond 20mins and is often not clinically noted. Es:Es leads to a prolonged block but is a very rare genotype (approx. 1:100,000). The more common genotype accounting for prolonged block is Ea:Ea, which has an incidence of 1:2800 and prolongs duration for over 2 hours. This is the most likely answer.

Hepatic disease is one of the causes of acquired plasma cholinesterase deficiency due to synthetic failure and can lead to prolongation of block. Other acquired factors include pregnancy, hyperthyroidism, cancer, and renal failure. Numerous drugs are also known to affect the duration of suxamethonium, e.g. procaine (competes with suxamethonium for pseudocholinesterase), lithium, and magnesium (potentiates the action of suxamethonium at the neuromuscular junction) and the oral contraceptive pill (reduces plasma cholinesterase activity by up to 20%). It is unlikely that any of these would prolong the effect for the 2 hours duration stated in the question.

Further reading

Peck TE, Hill SA, Williams M. *Pharmacology for Anaesthesia and Intensive Care*, 2nd edition. Greenwich Medical Media, 2003.

Smith S, Scarth E. *Drugs in Anaesthesia and Intensive Care*, 5th edition. Oxford University Press, 2016. Suxamethonium.

5. A

Atracurium clearance is little altered by hepatic or renal impairment. Its major metabolic pathway is Hofmann degradation, resulting in metabolites with insignificant neuromuscular blocking activity.

Renal impairment increases the clinical duration of action of mivacurium by a factor of 1.5, and hepatic impairment increases it by a factor of 3.

The pharmacokinetics of rocuronium are little altered by renal impairment. Hepatic impairment leads to a decreased clearance by 1 ml/kg/min, with a corresponding increase in the duration of action. Suxamethonium is readily hydrolysed by plasma cholinesterase at an *in vivo* rate of 3–7 mg/L/min. 2–10% of an administered dose is excreted unchanged in the urine. The half-life of vecuronium is prolonged in renal failure, in which 25–30% of a dose is excreted unchanged. However, this has no clinically significant increase in its duration of action.

Further reading

Smith S, Scarth E. *Drugs in Anaesthesia and Intensive Care*, 5th edition. Oxford University Press, 2016. Atracurium, Mivacurium, Rocuronium, Suxamethonium, Vecuronium.

6. E

Clearance is minimally altered by hepatic or renal impairment. Dosage adjustment is therefore unnecessary. In this patient's case raised transaminase levels may be associated with rhabdomyolysis and would not necessarily indicate hepatic impairment.

The onset of activity is likely to be lengthened in those receiving chronic anticonvulsant therapy, while the duration of action is shortened. As this patient requires a continuous infusion, this has less bearing. Its use appears to be safe in those susceptible to malignant hyperthermia and is not contraindicated in such cases.

Haemofiltration has a minimal effect on the plasma levels of atracurium or its metabolite, laudanosine. Given the use of continuous hemofiltration, this would be a key consideration in a patient requiring neuromuscular blockade for the management of ARDS.

Laudanosine, along with a quaternary monoacrylate, is a product of the major Hofmann degradative pathway. Hydrolysis via non-specific plasma esterases is its minor metabolic pathway, producing a quaternary alcohol and a quaternary acid. The C_{max} values of laudanosine are lower in patients receiving intravenous infusions of cisatracurium, compared with those receiving a continuous atracurium infusion. However, this would not necessarily guide its use.

Further reading

Smith S, Scarth E. *Drugs in Anaesthesia and Intensive Care*, 5th edition. Oxford University Press, 2016. Atracurium.

7. A

Edrophonium has a lesser duration of effect (10 minutes) compared to neostigmine (40–60 minutes). It does, however, have a more rapid onset to peak effect at 0.8–2 minutes, compared to neostigmine at 7–11 minutes following intravenous administration.

Neostigmine is up to 12–16 more potent than edrophonium. The intravenous dose of edrophonium for reversal of competitive neuromuscular blockade is 0.5–0.7 mg/kg, while that of neostigmine is 0.05–0.07 mg/kg. The muscarinic effects of the drug are correspondingly easier to counteract than those of neostigmine. This is important should a reversal of its effects be required with atropine.

Neostigmine is hydrolysed by acetylcholinesterase at a slower rate than acetylcholine. The metabolic pathway of edrophonium is uncertain. Resolution of weakness is noted following its administration in myasthenia. Its administration would potentiate a cholinergic crisis, thereby allowing differentiation between these presentations. Its binding to acetylcholinesterase is not a distinguishing feature. Edrophonium reversibly binds to the anionic site of acetylcholinesterase, while neostigmine binds to the esteratic site of acetylcholinesterase.

Further reading

Smith S, Scarth E. *Drugs in Anaesthesia and Intensive Care*, 5th edition. Oxford University Press, 2016. Edrophonium.

Chapter 5

Analgesics

Opioids

QUESTIONS

Multiple-Choice Questions

1. Effects of morphine include

A Bradycardia in high doses

B Miosis via stimulation of the Edinger–Westphal nucleus

C Decreased brainstem sensitivity to carbon dioxide compared to hypoxia

D Reduced common bile duct pressure

E Morphine decreases the secretion of antidiuretic hormone (ADH)

2. Regarding the metabolism of opioids

A Diamorphine must be metabolized to be active

B Metabolism of alfentanil is delayed by co-administration of midazolam

C Morphine is metabolized to morphine -6-glucuronide, which has active effects

D Remifentanil metabolism occurs in the liver by N-demethylation to nor-remifentanil

E The majority of codeine is excreted unchanged in the urine

3. Regarding drug passage across membranes

A Diamorphine is more lipid soluble compared to morphine

B Fentanyl has a faster onset of action compared to alfentanil

C Fentanyl is highly lipid soluble compared with alfentanil

D The higher the fraction of ionized drug the faster the onset

E The pKa value is dependent on whether the drug is acidic or basic

4. Regarding remifentanil

A Clearance is independent of renal and hepatic function

B Does not cause histamine release

C Has centrally mediated vagal activity

D Is a pure KOP (or Kappa) receptor agonist

E The administration of an anticholinergic drug will enhance the metabolism of remifentanil

5. Naloxone

A May alleviate pruritus following intrathecal administration of opioids

B Can be used in the treatment of clonidine overdose

C Is a competitive agonist to opioid receptors

D Is effective in the treatment of benzodiazepine overdose

E Is suitable for oral administration

6. Cardiovascular effects of opioids include

A Bradycardia of vagal origin

B A dose-dependent decrease in cardiac output

C A decrease in systemic vascular resistance

D A minimal to no effect on myocardial contractility

E Precipitation of arrhythmias

7. Tramadol

A Can safely be prescribed to patients on fluoxetine

B Inhibits reuptake of serotonin and enhances noradrenaline release

C Is a partial agonist to dopamine receptors

D Naloxone has no impact on the analgesic effects of tramadol

E Ultra-rapid metabolizers are more common in the Black compared with the white population

Single Best Answers

1. You are asked to review a ventilated intensive care unit (ICU) patient who is failing to wake despite their sedation being stopped. Prior to admission to hospital, they were found collapsed with a reduced level of consciousness. A collateral history is suggestive of a morphine overdose. Which of the following statements is correct?

A A transthoracic echocardiogram is likely to demonstrate a reduced left ventricular ejection fraction

B Adults are more sensitive to opioids compared to neonates due to higher levels of mu-receptor expression

C Morphine may precipitate coma in patients with hypopituitarism

D Oral ingestion of morphine is unlikely to be the cause of a reduced Glasgow Coma Scale (GCS)

E Use of haemodialysis will reduce the patient's time on a ventilator

2. You are asked to attend the emergency department to assist with the management of an intravenous drug user who has had a respiratory arrest. Drug paraphernalia consistent with opioid use was found at the scene. In considering the mechanism by which opioids may result in respiratory arrest, which of the following is most likely to have occurred?

A Opioids act through competitive enzyme inhibition

B Opioids exert their effect through the inhibition of Na channels, thereby hyperpolarizing cell membranes

C Opioids have an intracellular site of drug-receptor interaction

D Opioids increase potassium conductance, thereby hyperpolarizing cell membranes

E Opioids interact with receptors leading to alteration of DNA expression

3. You are asked to review a postoperative patient on the surgical ward. Two days ago, the patient had a revision total hip replacement. Spinal anaesthesia with morphine was performed and the patient had a propofol target-controlled infusion for deep sedation. The patient has a morphine patient-controlled analgesia (PCA) system attached which they have been using for the last two days. The PCA prescription settings are as follows: Bolus 1 mg, Lockout 5 minutes, Background zero. They have also been receiving oral paracetamol and ibuprofen. Her past medical history includes mild asthma. The patient is complaining of chest tightness, nausea, and itching, and is experiencing urinary urgency and hesitancy since her catheter was removed 12 hours ago. Which of the following is most likely to be correct?

A Bronchospasm is unlikely to be caused by morphine due to its immunoprotective properties

B Nausea caused by morphine is exclusively related to decreased gastrointestinal motility

C Prolonged use of morphine causes bladder irritability

D Reducing the rate of morphine administration can help limit histamine-induced bronchospasm

E The intrathecal route of administration precludes the development of pruritus

4. You are working in a chronic pain clinic. The patient you are reviewing has chronic lower limb pain following an industrial injury, after which they were unable to work. In addition to their chronic pain history, they also have generalized anxiety disorder and occasionally take diazepam for symptom control. They were originally referred to the clinic due to abuse of a prescribed slow-release morphine preparation and also oral morphine for breakthrough pain. However, following the instigation of an opioid withdrawal programme using methadone, they have now been successfully converted to alternative analgesia. Concerning the long-term use, dependence, and tolerance of opioids, which of the following is most likely to be correct?

A Chronic use of opioids will promote the development of further opioid receptors throughout the central nervous system

B Likelihood of receptor desensitization is greater when co-administered with benzodiazepines

C Methadone acts as a pure N-methyl-D-aspartate (NMDA) receptor antagonist

D Morphine can be tested for in the urine to check for abstinence

E Tolerance to opioids can develop following the first use

5. You are working on a maternity unit and have been asked to review a patient on the post-natal ward. The patient had a caesarean section two days ago and is complaining of postoperative pain and a new cough. You are reviewing her prescription chart and see that codeine phosphate has recently been prescribed as an antitussive. Concerning the use of codeine phosphate, which is most likely to be correct?

A All enzymes dependent on codeine metabolism display genetic polymorphism

B Analgesic effects are mediated through specific codeine receptors

C Codeine can be routinely used as analgesia for breastfeeding mothers

D Codeine has a low affinity for opioid receptors

E Codeine is approximately half as potent as morphine

6. You are about to anaesthetize a 28-year-old female patient who has a penetrating eye injury. A pregnancy test performed on the ward reveals she is in early pregnancy. Her past medical history is unremarkable, aside from currently taking erythromycin for otitis externa. You are considering your choice of induction agents which may include alfentanil. Regarding the use of alfentanil, which of the following is most likely to be correct?

A Alfentanil is highly lipid soluble thereby resulting in a fast onset of action

B Alfentanil is predominately albumin bound in the plasma

C Bolus dosing of the drug causes a temporary increase in intraocular pressure

D Concomitant use of erythromycin may significantly inhibit the clearance of alfentanil

E The molecular size of alfentanil prevents passage across the placenta

7. You have been asked to review a journal article for presentation at your department's weekly journal club. The paper relates to research on opioid receptors. Which of the following statements relating to opioid receptors is correct?

A Buprenorphine is an inverse agonist at MOP/mu receptor

B Dynorphin A is the endogenous ligand to the DOP receptor

C KOP/kappa receptor stimulation does not cause respiratory depression

D MOP/mu receptors are located specific to the spinal cord

E The NOP receptor produces the euphoric effects of opioids

ANSWERS

Multiple-Choice Questions

1. **TTTFF**

Morphine has minimal effects on the cardiovascular system, the predominant effect is orthostatic hypotension secondary to a decrease in system vascular resistance. It may cause bradycardia when administered in high doses. Miosis is produced as a result of stimulation of the Edinger–Westphal nucleus; this can be reversed by atropine. The principal respiratory effect of morphine is respiratory depression; it decreases the sensitivity of the brainstem to carbon dioxide, while the hypoxia response is less affected. Morphine increases the tone of ureters, bladder detrusor muscle, and sphincters, which can increase common bile duct pressure. Morphine increases the secretion of ADH and can lead to impaired water excretion and hyponatraemia.

Further reading

Peck T, Hill S, Williams M. *Pharmacology for Anaesthesia and Intensive Care*, 4th edition. Cambridge University Press, 2014. Pages 128–131.

Smith S, Scarth E. *Drugs in Anaesthesia and Intensive Care*, 5th edition. Oxford University Press, 2016. Morphine.

2. **TTTFF**

Diamorphine undergoes rapid enzymatic hydrolysis in the plasma to 6-0-acetylmorphine, which is the active form of the drug. Alfentanil is metabolized in the liver by N-dealkylation to noralfentanil. Cytochrome P450 3A3 and 3A4 play a predominant role in alfentanil metabolism and may be subject to competitive inhibition by the co-administration of midazolam. This can lead to the prolongation of the drug effects of midazolam and alfentanil. Morphine is metabolized in the liver to morphine-3-glucuronide, morphine-6-glucuronide, and normorphine. Morphine-6-glucuronide is more potent than morphine and has analgesic effects. Morphine-3-glucuronide has effects on arousal. The metabolism of remifentanil is unique among the opioid class; it undergoes rapid ester hydrolysis by non-specific plasma and tissue esterases to remifentanil acid, 4600-fold less potent than remifentanil. Codeine is extensively metabolized in the liver, and only a small proportion (5–15%) is excreted unchanged in the urine. There are three main mechanisms: by glucuronidation to codeine-6-glucuronide (10–20%); by N-demethylation to norcodeine (10–20%); and by O-demethylation to morphine (5–15%).

Further reading

Smith S, Scarth E. *Drugs in Anaesthesia and Intensive Care*, 5th edition. Oxford University Press, 2016. Alfentanil, Cisatracurium, Diamorphine, Esmolol, Remifentanil.

3. TFTFF

The cell membrane consists of a phospholipid bilayer, which is lipophilic in nature. Drugs which are weak acids or bases can exist in ionized/charged and unionized/uncharged forms depending on the pH of the environment it is exposed to. Only the unionized fraction of a drug is able to cross the lipophilic cell membrane. The higher the concentration of unionized drug present, the faster its onset of action will be. The pKa is the pH at which 50% of the drug is ionized; this value is dependent on the structure of the drug and not whether it is an acid or base. The pKa of alfentanil is 6.5; it is 89% unionized at pH of 7.4 and has a relatively low lipid solubility. Despite low lipid solubility, it has a faster onset of action compared to fentanyl due to this large, unionized fraction. Fentanyl has a much higher lipid solubility but a higher pKa of 8.4, with only 9% unionized at pH 7.4. Due to its higher lipid solubility, diamorphine has a faster onset of action than morphine.

Further reading

Peck T, Hill S, Williams M. *Pharmacology for Anaesthesia and Intensive Care*, 4th edition. Cambridge University Press, 2014. Factors influencing the rate of diffusion pp. 5–8, Alfentanil p. 136, Fentanyl p. 135.

Smith S, Scarth E. *Drugs in Anaesthesia and Intensive Care*, 5th edition. Oxford University Press, 2016. Diamorphine.

4. TTTFF

Remifentanil is a pure MOP agonist (or mu-agonist). The MOP receptor appears to be specifically involved in the mediation of analgesia and is located throughout the central nervous system. Remifentanil is present as a white lyophilized powder to be reconstituted before use. It has a pKa of 7.1 and is 68% unionized at a pH of 7.4. Remifentanil is metabolized rapidly by non-specific plasma esterase. The context-sensitive half-time is fixed due to the quantity of these esterases. The clearance is independent of renal and hepatic function. It does not cause histamine release but is associated with chest wall rigidity which may be related to MOP receptors on GABA-ergic interneurons. Remifentanil has centrally mediated vagal activity and can decrease heart rate by 20%. As reminfentanil's metabolism is independent of the plasma cholinesterase system, the administration of anticholinesterase drugs will not affect it.

Further reading

Smith S, Scarth E. *Drugs in Anaesthesia and Intensive Care*, 5th edition. Oxford University Press, 2016. Remifentanil.

5. TTFFF

Naloxone is a substituted oxymorphone derivative. It is a competitive antagonist at mu-, delta-, kappa-, and sigma-opioid receptors. It has the highest affinity for mu receptors. It is used for the reversal of respiratory depression due to opioids and can also be used in the treatment of clonidine overdose. Mu-receptor antagonists have been shown to have antipruritic effects. Results on the efficacy of naloxone for treating opioid-induced pruritus have been mixed but some studies show a positive benefit. It is not effective in the treatment of benzodiazepine overdose; this is flumazenil. Naloxone will precipitate acute withdrawal symptoms in opioid addicts. It may be administered intravenously, intramuscularly, or subcutaneously. It is 91% absorbed when administered orally but has an oral bioavailability of 2% due to extensive first-pass metabolism. It has a duration of effect that may be shorter than the opioid it is intended to treat, additional doses may be necessary.

Further reading

Kumar K, Singh SI. Neuraxial opioid-induced pruritus: an update. *J Anaesthesiol Clin Pharmacol*, 2013;29(3):303–307.

Smith S, Scarth E. *Drugs in Anaesthesia and Intensive Care*, 5th edition. Oxford University Press, 2016. Naloxone.

6. TFTTF

Overall, opioids have minimal effects on the cardiovascular system when used in normal doses. High doses of opioids, particularly remifentanil, will cause bradycardia, which is vagal in origin. Alfentanil and fentanyl will obtund the cardiovascular response to laryngoscopy and intubation. Opioids can cause a decrease in systemic vascular resistance, partly mediated by histamine release and a reduction in sympathetic tone. They do not have direct myocardial depressant effects and do not cause a dose-dependent decrease in cardiac output. They are drugs not commonly associated with arrhythmia generation.

Further reading

Gupta A, Singh-Radcliff N. *Pharmacology in Anesthesia Practice*, 1st edition. Oxford University Press, 2013. Chapter 3.1 Opioids.

7. FFFFT

Tramadol is a cyclohexanol derivative. It is a racemic mixture of two enantiomers, with their own specific actions. It is a non-selective agonist at mu-, kappa-, and delta opioid receptors. It also inhibits neural reuptake of norepinephrine and enhances serotonin release. Its main action is centrally mediated analgesia, partly through the activation of descending serotonergic and noradrenergic pathways. Naloxone will partially reverse the analgesic effect of tramadol by 30%, but has been rarely reported associated with long-term administration. Tramadol is metabolized by CYP2D6 and CYP3A4. Several selective serotonin reuptake inhibitors (SSRIs), including fluoxetine, are moderate-potent inhibitors of CYP2D6 and hence lead to increased tramadol concentrations. Co-administration also increases the risk of serotonin syndrome. Other drugs that should be avoided include monoamine oxidase inhibitors. Serotonin syndrome is characterized by features including neuromuscular hyperactivity, autonomic dysfunction, and altered mental state. Severe toxicity is a medical emergency.

The prevalence of ultra-rapid metabolizers (a genetic variant of CYP2D6) has been quoted at 29% in the African (especially Ethiopian) population compared to 3.5–6.5% in white people. Ultra-rapid metabolizers can lead to a sudden peak in O-desmethyltramadol (M1) which is pharmacologically active and has a higher affinity for opioid receptors compared to the parent drug.

Further reading

Smith S, Scarth E. *Drugs in Anaesthesia and Intensive Care*, 5th edition. Oxford University Press, 2016. Tramadol.

Single Best Answers

1. C

Morphine inhibits the release of adrenocorticotrophic hormone, prolactin, and gonadotrophic hormones. The use of this drug in patients with hypopituitarism may, therefore, precipitate coma. Neonates are more sensitive than adults to morphine due to immature liver enzymes and a reduced conjugating capacity, therefore, corresponding dose reduction is necessary. Morphine has minimal effects on the cardiovascular system but its anxiolytic and vasodilatory effects are used as a treatment in left ventricular failure. Morphine cannot be removed by haemodialysis or peritoneal dialysis. The drug is well absorbed orally, due to extensive first-pass metabolism. The bioavailability via this route is 15–50%.

Further reading

Peck T, Hill S, Williams M. *Pharmacology for Anaesthesia and Intensive Care*, 4th edition. Cambridge University Press, 2014. Morphine pp. 128–131.

Smith S, Scarth E. *Drugs in Anaesthesia and Intensive Care*, 5th edition. Oxford University Press, 2016. Morphine.

2. D

Opioids interact as agonists with one or several specific opioid receptors: the mu-, kappa-, delta-, and NOP receptors. They are membrane-spanning receptors that are linked to inhibitory G proteins (Gi). The following sequence occurs: drug interaction with presynaptic Gi-protein receptors; closure of voltage-sensitive calcium channels, which leads to an increase in intracellular calcium concentration. In turn, this causes increased potassium conductance and hyperpolarization of the membrane by potassium efflux. This leads to adenylate cyclase inhibition and reduced levels of cAMP. The overall effect is a decrease in membrane excitability that results in the inhibition of transmitter release between nerve cells.

Further reading

Peck T, Hill S, Williams M. *Pharmacology for Anaesthesia and Intensive Care*, 4th edition. Cambridge University Press, 2014. Opioids and related drugs pp. 127–128.

Smith S, Scarth E. *Drugs in Anaesthesia and Intensive Care*, 5th edition. Oxford University Press, 2016. Morphine.

3. D

There is some evidence to show that opioids can decrease macrophage and T-cell activity, but they do not exhibit immunoprotective properties. A common side effect of opioids is nausea and vomiting—this is in part centrally mediated due to stimulation of the chemo receptor trigger zone via dopamine and 5-HT receptors. Opioids increase the tone of ureters, bladder detrusor muscle, and sphincter, and may lead to urinary retention rather than irritability. Morphine results in the release of histamine which may lead to bronchoconstriction, rash, and pruritus. Reducing the rate of administration of the drug may help to limit bronchospasm. Development of pruritus is most marked following intrathecal and epidural administration.

Further reading

Gupta A, Singh-Radcliff N. *Pharmacology in Anesthesia Practice*, 1st edition. Oxford University Press, 2013. Chapter 3.1 Opioids.

Peck T, Hill S, Williams M. *Pharmacology for Anaesthesia and Intensive Care*, 4th edition. Cambridge University Press, 2014. Morphine pp. 128–131.

Smith S, Scarth E. *Drugs in Anaesthesia and Intensive Care*, 5th edition. Oxford University Press, 2016. Morphine.

4. D

Opioids exhibit the phenomenon of tolerance; whereby chronic use will lead to altered sensitivity of receptors so that over time larger doses of the drug will be required to produce the same pharmacological effect. This will not occur after first use of the drug. Greater numbers of receptors are not developed following chronic use. Desensitization refers to chronic loss of receptor response over time; benzodiazepines have no effect on this. Methadone is an opioid with a high affinity for mu receptors. Due to its high oral bioavailability (75%) and long plasma half-life, it is used in the treatment process of intravenous opioid addicts. It may also act as an antagonist at NMDA receptors and has a possible role in the treatment of neuropathic pain. Metabolites of opioids, rather than the parent drug, are removed via renal clearance and their presence can be detected for in urine analysis.

Further reading

Peck T, Hill S, Williams M. *Pharmacology for Anaesthesia and Intensive Care*, 4th edition. Cambridge University Press, 2014. Tachyphylaxis, desensitization and tolerance pp. 38–39, Methadone p. 139.

5. D

Codeine is a methylated morphine derivative with a very low affinity for opioid receptors. It acts as a prodrug for morphine and it is this morphine metabolite which is responsible for the analgesic effects. The antitussive effects of codeine are due to interaction with high-affinity specific codeine receptors. Approximately 10% of codeine is metabolized to morphine and it is ten times less potent than morphine, not half. Codeine is metabolized in the liver via three main pathways.

The cytochrome P450 enzyme, CYP2D6, which is responsible for the conversion to morphine, exhibits genetic variability; fast metabolizers produce more morphine. Poor metabolizers experience few analgesic effects. Codeine is not recommended for use in breastfeeding (BNF).

Further reading

NICE. Codeine Phosphate, 2022. Available at: https://bnf.nice.org.uk/drug/codeine-phosphate.html

Smith S, Scarth E. *Drugs in Anaesthesia and Intensive Care*, 5th edition. Oxford University Press, 2016. Codeine.

6. D

Alfentanil is a potent mu-receptor agonist. Cytochrome P450 3A3 and 3A4 play a predominant role in metabolism and these enzymes may be subject to competitive inhibition by other drugs. Erythromycin may reduce the clearance of alfentanil by inhibition of hepatic CYP450. Alfentanil may lower intraocular pressure by approximately 45%. Alfentanil has a relatively low lipid solubility, although the onset of action is fast due to the large unionized proportion at physiological pH. Alfentanil is 85–92% protein bound, predominately to alpha-1 acid glycoprotein, with a volume of distribution of 0.4–1 l /kg. It will cross the placenta. Due to a small volume of distribution and short elimination half-life, a single dose has a relatively short duration of action.

Further reading

Smith S, Scarth E. Drugs in Anaesthesia and Intensive Care, 5th edition. Oxford University Press, 2016. Alfentanil.

7. C

Dynorphin A is the endogenous ligand for the KOP receptor, not the DOP receptor (this is Leu- or Met-enkephalin). Buprenorphine is a partial agonist at meu receptors, from which it dissociates slowly, leading to prolonged analgesic effects. The stimulation of specifically KOP/kappa receptors does not cause respiratory depression. However, KOP/kappa agonists appear to have some antagonistic effects on mu receptors which limits their clinical usefulness. The mu receptors are found throughout the central nervous system and are not exclusive to the spinal cord. The majority are located presynaptically in the periaqueductal grey and in the dorsal horn of the spinal cord. They are also present in the cerebral cortex. Stimulation of the mu receptors will mediate analgesia as well as many of the side effects associated with opioids, including respiratory depression and constipation. The euphoric effects of opioids are also mediated through the MOP/mu receptor.

Further reading

McDonald J, Lambert DG. Opioid receptors. *Cont Educ Anaesth Crit Care Pain*, 2015;15(5):219–224.

Peck T, Hill S, Williams M. *Pharmacology for Anaesthesia and Intensive Care*, 4th edition. Cambridge University Press, 2014. Opioids and related drugs pp. 127–128.

Analgesics

Non-opioids

QUESTIONS

Multiple-Choice Questions

1. Carbamazepine

A Is the first-line agent used when a diagnosis of trigeminal neuralgia is suspected

B Rashes occur in 3% of patients

C Is excreted unchanged in the urine

D Is pro-arrhythmogenic

E Regular monitoring of hepatic function is required for patients taking long-term carbamazepine therapy

2. Ketamine

A Is a non-competitive agonist of the N-methyl-D-aspartate (NMDA) receptor Ca^{2+} channel pore

B Its action results in an increase of presynaptic glutamate

C In higher doses, has some local anaesthetic activity

D Is a racemic mixture, which has benefits for use in patients with bronchospasm

E Reduces salivary secretions

3. Clonidine

A Reduces cardiac contractility and cardiac output

B Is an alpha-2 agonist

C Is indicated for use in migraine

D The analgesic effector site is the dorsal horn of the spinal cord

E Increases blood pressure

4. Paracetamol

A The mechanism of action of paracetamol is poorly understood, but there is evidence of action involving prostaglandin synthesis, serotonergic, and cannabinoid pathways

B The antipyretic effects are thought to be secondary to antagonism of prostaglandin E within the central nervous system

C 5% of patients expressing an aspirin allergy have a cross-sensitivity to paracetamol

D Is metabolized to N-acetyl-p-benzo-quinoneimine (NAPQI), which is then activated by glutathione conjugation

E Is not removed by haemodialysis

5. Non-steroidal anti-inflammatory drugs (NSAIDs)

A 35% of a diclofenac dose is excreted in bile

B Use of NSAIDs results in reduced platelet aggregation and prolonged bleeding time

C Ibuprofen has no effect on foetal circulation if administered maternally

D Ibuprofen causes bronchoconstriction in 20% of patients suffering from asthma

E There is an association between prolonged use of NSAIDs and arterial thrombotic events in patients with cardiovascular disease

6. Tramadol

A Has agonist effects at multiple opioid receptors and enhances serotonin release centrally

B Can often be effective in managing postoperative shivering

C Is a racemic mixture of two enantiomers

D Enhances neuronal noradrenaline reuptake

E The analgesic effects of tramadol are fully reversed by naloxone

7. Gabapentin

A Is an antineuropathic analgesic

B Is a gamma-aminobutyric acid (GABA) antagonist

C Stimulates glutamate decarboxylase

D Has an oral bioavailability of 40%

E Is removed by haemodialysis

Single Best Answers

1.
A patient is given analgesic 'Z'. They experience tachycardia, nausea, rash, and an increase in salivary secretions.

Which drug are they most likely to have been given?

A Amitriptyline

B Duloxetine

C Ketamine

D Magnesium

E Pregabalin

2.
A female 68-year-old 85 kg patient is prescribed a lidocaine infusion at 3 mg/kg to be administered intravenously over 90 minutes.

Which of the following statements is the most accurate?

A A blood level of 6µg/ml is below the expected threshold for central nervous system toxicity

B A patient with chronic hypercarbia will be at higher risk of lidocaine central nervous system toxicity, so doses should be reduced

C Co-administration of a drug that increases hepatic blood flow may require lidocaine dose to be reduced

D Doses can be increased by 25% in patients with moderate heart failure due to their increased volume of distribution

E Dosing should be based on a patient's lean body weight

3. A patient who is regularly on amitriptyline is given prochlorperazine. You are urgently called to review the patient. They have a blood pressure of 50//30 and a heart rate of 140. Another anaesthetist attends to the patient with you and slowly administers a 250 mcg dose of diluted adrenaline intravenously. The patient's blood pressure now becomes unrecordable.

Which of the following statements is the most appropriate explanation?

A Insufficient adrenaline has been given to the patient

B Prochlorperazine and amitriptyline have physically precipitated

C Prochlorperazine blocks alpha-2 receptors

D Procyclidine should have been given to the patient before adrenaline administered

E There is unopposed beta2 receptor agonism

4. You are told the following information about a drug:

• Site of action: alpha-2-delta subunit of voltage-gated calcium channels
• Bioavailability of 60% declines with increasing doses
• Not bound to plasma proteins
• Side effects include weight gain

Which drug is this most likely to be?

A Flunarizine

B Gabapentin

C Nimodipine

D Pregabalin

E Ziconotide

5. Regarding capsaicin—who is the least suitable to use this medication?

A An asthmatic patient with idiopathic trigeminal neuralgia

B A diabetic patient with painful neuropathy

C A patient with renal impairment (eGFR 35) and peripheral neuropathic pain

D A patient with severe liver disease seeking symptomatic relief from osteoarthritis

E A pregnant patient with post-herpetic neuralgia

6. You are prescribing nefopam to a patient during an acute pain ward round. The medical student with you asks you to tell them more about the drug.

Which of the following statements concerning nefopam is most accurate?

A It is a benzodiazepine

B Its analgesic potency is approximately one-tenth of that of morphine

C Mechanism of action involves GABA receptors

D Patients should be warned of the side effect of sweating

E Respiratory depression is associated with this drug

7. You are prescribing intravenous clonidine to a patient on the intensive care unit.

Which of the following statements best describes clonidine's cardiovascular effects?

A Antagonism of vascular alpha-2 adrenoceptors

B Decreases vagal tone

C Progressively increases the responsiveness of peripheral vessels to other vasoactive substances

D Reduces cardiac contractility

E Reduces noradrenaline release

ANSWERS

Multiple-Choice Questions

1. TTFFT

Carbamazepine is the first-choice analgesic in pharmacological treatment of trigeminal neuralgia. Rashes occur in up to 3% of patients. Carbamazepine undergoes hepatic oxidative metabolism to an epoxide. In chronic use, carbamazepine is a hepatic enzyme-inducer, inducing its own metabolism. This 'inducing effect' also results in reduced plasma concentrations of other medications that rely on hepatic metabolism. Carbamazepine has antiarrhythmic properties and depresses atrioventricular node conduction. Chronic carbamazepine therapy can result in hepatic dysfunction as well as mild neutropenia and rarely aplastic anaemia. Regular monitoring is therefore essential.

Further reading

Smith S, Scarth E. *Drugs in Anaesthesia and Intensive Care*, 5th edition. Oxford University Press, 2016. Carbamazepine.

2. FFTTF

Ketamine is a non-competitive antagonist of the NMDA receptor Ca^{2+} channel pore. The use of ketamine results in reduced concentrations of presynaptic glutamate, therefore reducing the onward progression of action potentials in the pain pathway. There are also complex interactions with opioid receptors. Ketamine is a racemic mixture of S-[+]-Ketamine and R-[–]-Ketamine in equal proportions. The S-[+]-Ketamine enantiomer has four times the affinity for the NMDA receptor compared to the R-[–]-Ketamine enantiomer. However, the R-[–]-Ketamine enantiomer has greater action on bronchial smooth muscle relaxation by reducing acetylcholine-mediation smooth muscle contraction. Ketamine increases salivary secretions and therefore an antisialogogue medication is usually used concomitantly.

Further reading

Smith S, Scarth E. *Drugs in Anaesthesia and Intensive Care*, 5th edition. Oxford University Press, 2016. Ketamine.

3. FTTTT

Clonidine has no effect on cardiac contractility and maintains cardiac output. The effects of clonidine are mainly due to the alpha-2 agonist actions, reducing noradrenaline release from sympathetic nerve terminals resulting in lower sympathetic tone and reduced blood pressure. However, initially clonidine causes a hypertensive response secondary to the activation of vascular alpha-1 receptors. In parallel, vagal tone is also increased. Chronic low-dose clonidine is indicated in migraine prophylaxis; its mechanism of action being the reduction in responsiveness to vasoactive and sympathetic stimulation, resulting in reduced vascular spasm. However, its use has been superseded by other forms of migraine prophylaxis and is no longer commonly used. Total discontinuation of clonidine risks potentially life-threatening rebound hypertension and tachycardia.

Further reading

Smith S, Scarth E. *Drugs in Anaesthesia and Intensive Care*, 5th edition. Oxford University Press, 2016. Clonidine.

4. TTTFF

Paracetamol is polymodal in its mechanisms of action. As well as the COX-1 and COX-2 isoenzyme inhibition, serotonergic, and endocannabinoid antagonism, paracetamol also inhibits peripheral bradykinin-sensitive chemoreceptors. This results in reduced primary afferent nociceptive impulse generation. Paracetamol is hepatically metabolized to glucuronide (60–80%), sulphate (20–30%), and 10% by CYP2E1 enzymes to a highly hepatotoxic intermediate metabolite N-acetyl-p-benzo-quinoneimine (NAPQI). NAPQI is then conjugated with glutathione, rendering it inactive. 1–5% of paracetamol is excreted unchanged in the urine. Paracetamol is removed by haemodialysis.

Further reading

Smith S, Scarth E. *Drugs in Anaesthesia and Intensive Care*, 5th edition. Oxford University Press, 2016. Paracetamol.

5. TTFTT

Diclofenac is a non-specific cyclo-oxygenase inhibitor. It is hepatically metabolized. Approximately 65% is excreted renally and 35% is excreted in bile.

Ibuprofen is also a non-specific COX inhibitor thus stopping the conversion of arachidonic acid to endoperoxidases and preventing the formation of thromboxanes, prostaglandins, and prostacyclin. Thromboxanes are critical in clotting due to local platelet activation and platelet aggregation.

Ibuprofen can trigger premature closure of the otherwise patent ductus arteriosus if administered during the third trimester of pregnancy.

Reduced production of the bronchodilator PGE_2 results in bronchoconstriction due to unopposed PGD_2 and $PGF_2\alpha$.

Further reading

Bennett A. The importance of COX-2 inhibition for aspirin induced asthma. *Thorax*, 2000;55(suppl 2):S54–S56.

Smith S, Scarth E. *Drugs in Anaesthesia and Intensive Care*, 5th edition. Oxford University Press, 2016. Diclofenac, Ibuprofen, Ketorolac.

6. TTTFF

Tramadol has antagonistic effects at mu-, kappa-, and delta-opioid receptors. It has a higher relative affinity for mu receptors. Other analgesic mechanisms of action include enhanced serotonin release and reduced noradrenaline reuptake. This increases the effectiveness of the descending pain pathways resulting in greater inhibition of ascending pain signals. Naloxone only reverses approximately 30% of the analgesia provided by tramadol. This is likely due to the multimodal analgesic activity of tramadol.

Further reading

Smith S, Scarth E. *Drugs in Anaesthesia and Intensive Care*, 5th edition. Oxford University Press, 2016. Tramadol.

7. TFTFT

Gabapentin, along with pregabalin, are analgesics used in a range of neuropathic pain conditions including painful diabetic neuropathy and post-herpetic neuralgia. Although structurally similar to the inhibitory neurotransmitter molecule GABA, the mechanism of action of gabapentin is one of antagonism of the alpha-2-delta subunit of the neuronal voltage-gated calcium channels.

Gabapentin stimulates glutamate decarboxylase resulting in greater levels of GABA conversion from glutamate. Higher levels of GABA result in reduced neuronal excitability because the neuronal threshold potential is not reached, reducing action potential propagation. Gabapentin has an oral bioavailability of 60%.

Further reading

Smith S, Scarth E. *Drugs in Anaesthesia and Intensive Care*, 5th edition. Oxford University Press, 2016. Gabapentin.

Single Best Answers

1. C

Ketamine is a non-competitive NMDA antagonist. Commonly associated side effects include increased saliva, transient rash (15%), postoperative nausea, and vomiting. Cardiovascular effects include tachycardia and hypertension due to increased sympathetic tone. Emergence delirium and hallucinations are also well-recognized side effects. Amitriptyline (a tricyclic antidepressant), duloxetine (a selective serotonin and noradrenaline reuptake inhibitor—'SNRI'), and pregabalin (a 'gabapentinoid') are all associated with a dry mouth in their side effect profiles. In addition to its uses in severe asthma, cardiac arrhythmias, pre-eclampsia/eclampsia, and electrolyte correction/nutrition, etc., magnesium has also been used as an analgesic. Side effects other than mild gastrointestinal upset are rare unless overdose or toxicity results.

Further reading

Smith S, Scarth E. *Drugs in Anaesthesia and Intensive Care*, 5th edition. Oxford University Press, 2016. Clonidine.

2. B

Although respiratory acidosis might be thought to reduce the risk of central nervous system toxicity with lidocaine (due to acidosis reducing unionized fraction of lidocaine) it has actually been shown that hypercarbia reduces lidocaine binding to plasma proteins and thereby increases the free fraction of the drug. Conversely, hypocarbia increases protein binding.

Therapeutic plasma levels are quoted as 2.5–3.5µg/ml and central nervous system toxicity can occur at 5µg/ml hence lidocaine has a narrow therapeutic index. Locally determined dosing protocols vary but doses should be appropriately reduced in patients with heart failure, severe liver disease, low plasma proteins and any situation which results in decreased hepatic blood flow (e.g. drugs, increasing age). Lidocaine has a high hepatic extraction ratio and has two active metabolites that have been associated with toxicity (monoethylglycyxylidide [MGEX] and glycylxylidide [GX]). Dosing should be based on adjusted body weight = ideal body weight + 0.4 (actual body weight – ideal body weight).

Lidocaine is an amide local anaesthetic that also has benefit as a systemic analgesic. It has been used by infusion to help manage chronic neuropathic pain and also in the context of acute postoperative pain as an antihyperalgesic agent. The strength of evidence of outcomes in acute pain literature is limited by small studies and much heterogeneity. Its mechanism of action as a systemic analgesic is thought to involve a reduction in the neo-proliferation of sodium channels, reduced inflammatory markers, reduced central sensitization, and decreased NMDA post-synaptic signalling.

Further reading

Budiansky AS, Margarson MP, Eipe N. Acute pain management in morbid obesity—an evidence-based clinical update. *Surg Obesity & Rel Dis*, 2017;13(3):523–532.

Eipe N, Gupta S, Penning J. Intravenous lidocaine for acute pain: an evidence-based clinical update. *BJA Education*, 2016;16(9):292–298.

Smith S, Scarth E. *Drugs in Anaesthesia and Intensive Care*, 5th edition. Oxford University Press, 2016. Lidocaine.

3. E

Phenothiazines (e.g. prochlorperazine) displace tricyclics from their plasma protein binding sites, thus increasing their activity. In high doses, amitriptyline can cause dysrhythmias (prolongs AV node conduction), profound hypotension, and tachycardia. Adrenaline in this circumstance could induce potentially fatal ventricular arrhythmias and in the context of amitriptyline should generally be avoided due to the risk of exaggerated hypertension (due to the noradrenaline reuptake inhibition from the amitriptyline).

However, with phenothiazines also involved the interaction is more complex; in addition to the above displacement effects, phenothiazines will block alpha-1 adrenoceptors that can lead to 'reversed adrenaline response'. Due to the blocked alpha-1 receptors, adrenaline's action on beta-2 receptors is relatively unopposed—this triggers vasodilatation in skeletal muscle arterioles further lowering blood pressure and leading to a refractory picture. Procyclidine blocks central cholinergic receptors and is used to treat extra-pyramidal symptoms, oculogyric crises, and Parkinson's disease.

Further reading

Smith S, Scarth E. *Drugs in Anaesthesia and Intensive Care*, 5th edition. Oxford University Press, 2016. Amitriptyline, Prochlorperazine.

4. B

Gabapentin is structurally related to GABA but doesn't interact with the GABA receptor—instead, it is the alpha-2-delta subunit of voltage-gated calcium channels which is the site of action. Pregabalin also has this site of action, but its bioavailability exceeds 90% and is independent of the administered dose. Weight gain has been associated with gabapentin, pregabalin, and flunarizine.

Flunarizine is a selective calcium channel blocker which has been used in the treatment of migraine and vertigo. Its bioavailability is >80%. Nimodipine is most frequently associated with the treatment of cerebral vasospasm and migraine. It has low bioavailability (<30%) and is highly protein bound. Some studies have indicated that while it does not have analgesic action by itself, it may potentiate an enhanced analgesic effect when combined with morphine or fentanyl. Ziconotide selectively blocks N-type calcium channel on A-delta and C fibres in the dorsal horn of the spinal cord. It has been intrathecally administered for refractory chronic pain and has a potency 1000 times greater than morphine.

Further reading

Smith S, Scarth E. *Drugs in Anaesthesia and Intensive Care*, 5th edition. Oxford University Press, 2016. Gabapentin, Nimodipine, Pregabalin.

5. A

Capsaicin (a chilli pepper extract) is an exogenous agonist at the TRPV1 vanilloid receptor which is selectively expressed on nociceptive fibres. This receptor is activated by extreme acidosis (pH <6) and heat (>43°C) but in combination, lower levels of stimuli can achieve activation. Endogenous agonists have also been determined including some leukotrienes and fatty acids. Activation of the receptor triggers the perception of burn, sting, or itch by the brain. Exposure to capsaicin results in a persistent, overwhelming biological signal which can defunctionalize nociceptive cell mitochondria, leads to loss of epidermal nerve fibres, and give long-lasting pain relief. Compliance with application can be improved by pretreatment with local anaesthetic creams.

Current UK indications for capsaicin are osteoarthritis, post-herpetic neuralgia, painful diabetic neuropathy (under expert supervision), and peripheral neuropathic pain. This is due to its topical application and thus very low systemic absorption which reduces the risk of systemic side effects. Although the safety of capsaicin in pregnancy has not been formally established, the consensus is that it is unlikely to cause adverse effects. It should not be used on broken skin.

No adjustments are required for renal or hepatic impairment. Some studies have highlighted asthma as a relative contraindication to capsaicin use due to a hypothesized increase in endovallinoids and thus TRV1 receptors in the airways of asthmatics, which may lead to symptom exacerbation.

Further reading

Anand P, Bley K. Topical capsaicin for pain management: therapeutic potential and mechanisms of action of the new high-concentration capsaicin 8% patch. Br J Anaesth, 2011;107(4):490–502.

6. D

Nefopam is a centrally acting non-opioid analgesic. It is a cyclic analogue of diphenhydramine and was initially developed as a muscle relaxant and antidepressant drug. The mechanism of action, although not fully elucidated, involves reuptake inhibition of serotonin, noradrenaline, and dopamine. It is also thought to interact with glutamate receptors. Nefopam is a racemic mixture; (+) nefopam is considerably more antinociceptive than (−) nefopam. First-pass metabolism is extensive. Metabolism is hepatic, with only 5% being excreted unchanged in urine. Respiratory depression is not a feature. Sweating is a relatively commonly reported side effect, along with nausea and drowsiness. Pharmacologically nefopam has been suggested to be ten times more potent than aspirin and equianalgesic to diclofenac. Some studies have reported 20 mg nefopam to be equipotent to 12 mg morphine and its use in the management of post-surgical pain has been estimated to reduce morphine consumption by approximately 30%.

Further reading

Evans MS, Lysakowski C, Tramèr MR. Nefopam for the prevention of postoperative pain: quantitative systematic review. BJA: Br J Anaesth, 2008;101(5):610–617.

Kim KH, Abdi S. Rediscovery of nefopam for the treatment of neuropathic pain. Korean J Pain, 2014;27(2):103–111.

7. E

Clonidine is an alpha agonist. It has actions on both α_1 and α_2 receptors with a 200:1 affinity for α_2. α_2 actions result in the stimulation of pre-synaptic receptors thus decreasing noradrenaline release from synaptic terminals. This reduces sympathetic tone and thereby increases vagal tone. Cardiac contractility is unaffected but systematic and coronary vascular resistance falls. It is common to see a transient increase in blood pressure on initial administration due to α_1 stimulation, but clinically this is followed by a sustained decrease in blood pressure. Heart rate typically reduces slightly with clonidine use. An analgesic mechanism involves α_2 adrenoceptor agonism both centrally at a spinal and supraspinal level, leading to descending modulation, dorsal horn inhibition of nociceptive neurons, and release of substance P.

Further reading

Smith S, Scarth E. *Drugs in Anaesthesia and Intensive Care*, 5th edition. Oxford University Press, 2016. Clonidine.

Antimicrobial agents

QUESTIONS

Multiple-Choice Questions

1. Amphotericin

A Is a mixture of two macrolides produced by *Streptomyces nodosus*

B Is only active against *Candida albicans*

C Binds to ribosomes thereby inhibiting fungal protein synthesis

D Use is associated with renal impairment

E Is well absorbed from the gastrointestinal (GI) tract

2. Oseltamivir

A Is active against the varicella-zoster virus

B Inhibits influenza A neuraminidase but not influenza B

C When administered orally, at least 75% of the dose reaches the systemic circulation as oseltamivir

D Exhibits high protein binding

E Resistance requires previous exposure to the drug

3. Fluoroquinolones

A Are derived from nalidixic acid

B Inhibits bacterial ribosomal proteins

C Are associated with tendon rupture

D May be used to treat *Yersinia pestis* infection

E May be used for post-exposure prophylaxis (PEP) against potential bioterrorism organisms

4. Caspofungin

A Is derived from phencyclidine
B Has high oral bioavailability
C Inhibits mammalian beta (1,3)-D-glucan
D Is highly protein bound
E Inhibits cytochrome P450

5. Aciclovir

A Is active against Sars-CoV-2
B Inhibits mammalian deoxyribonucleic acid polymerase
C Is activated by viral-coded thymidine kinase
D Is excreted by passive tubular filtration into the urine mostly unchanged
E Dosing should be reduced in renal impairment

6. Carbapenems

A Bind to penicillin-binding proteins within the bacterial cytoplasm
B Are available as oral preparations
C Exhibit low plasma protein binding
D Are active against anaerobic bacteria
E May be associated with seizure activity

7. Aminoglycosides

A Are not available in tablet form
B Are active against anaerobic bacteria
C Reversibly bind to specific bacterial ribosomal proteins (30S subunit)
D Reduce the action of non-depolarizing muscle relaxants
E Can be used safely in patients with myasthenia gravis

Single Best Answers

1. A 36-year-old woman is admitted to the intensive care unit (ICU) for vasoactive support following a diagnosis of likely septic shock. She is currently undergoing chemotherapy for carcinoma of the breast. Pertinent findings on clinical examination include a core temperature of 38.9°C and occasional rigors. Her chest is clear and abdominal examination is unremarkable. Cardiovascular examination reveals a tachycardia of 136 bpm and a non-invasive blood pressure of 76/57. An indwelling peripherally inserted central catheter (PICC) line, with some erythema at the insertion site, and peripheral cannula are noted. She also has an area on her right thigh, which is hot, erythematous, and painful to touch. A full blood count (FBC) reveals a neutrophil count of 0.3 × 10⁹ per litre. As part of her cancer treatment regimen, she is receiving G-CSF injections and ciprofloxacin. Blood cultures have been taken from the PICC line and also peripherally.

The next most appropriate course of action is:

A Administration of an additional dose of G-CSF together with an intravenous dose of ciprofloxacin (identical to the oral dose already taken by the patient)

B Administration of 2 g flucloxacillin intravenously, as an opportunistic skin commensal organism is the most likely septic focus of infection

C An intravenous dose of piperacillin with tazobactam with or without an aminoglycoside should be administered

D An intravenous dose of piperacillin with tazobactam with or without an aminoglycoside should be administered together with an intravenous dose of G-CSF

E Removal of the PICC line and administration of an empiric glycopeptide such as teicoplanin, as line sepsis is the most likely septic focus of infection

2. You are asked to review a previously fit and well 65-year-old man who is acutely unwell in the emergency department. A diagnosis of a lower respiratory tract infection has been made. Pertinent findings on clinical examination include a respiratory rate of 35 breaths per minute and a non-invasive blood pressure of 84/62. He is receiving oxygen via a non-rebreathe mask. A semi-recumbent anterior-posterior (AP) chest X-ray reveals some loss of the right heart border. Blood tests have been taken including blood cultures.

Regarding this patient's antimicrobial therapy, the next most appropriate course of action is:

A Administration of a macrolide antibiotic for five days

B Administration of a macrolide antibiotic for seven days

C Administration of a macrolide and a beta-lactamase stable penicillin-based antibiotic for at least seven days

D Administration of a macrolide and penicillin-based antibiotic for five days

E Administration of a macrolide and penicillin-based antibiotic for seven to ten days

3. A 41-year-old woman is admitted to ICU via the cardiac catheter lab having undergone an emergency angiogram for a suspected acute ST-segment elevation myocardial infarction. No coronary intervention has been performed. She has a Glasgow Coma Scale (GCS) of 15/15 but has been transferred to ICU as she is requiring low-dose vasoactive support. A presumptive diagnosis of viral myocarditis has been made.

Regarding this patient's antiviral therapy, the next most appropriate course of action is:

A Administration of entecavir with best supportive care

B Administration of foscarnet with best supportive care

C Administration of oseltamivir with best supportive care

D Administration of ribavirin with best supportive care

E Best supportive care but no antiviral agent

4. A 62-year-old female patient is on your ICU. She was admitted several days ago as being non-specifically unwell, reported weight loss, and electrolyte derangements were detected on blood tests precipitating ICU admission for central venous access correction. A chest X-ray revealed multiple soft tissue densities throughout both lung fields. On further questioning, she reports recently working in sub-Saharan Africa at a school in a rural area and was given 'anti-TB medication' to protect her. She has no visible Bacillus Calmette–Guérin (BCG) scar. A diagnosis of TB has been made with resistance to isoniazid.

The next most appropriate course of action is:

A Start rifampicin, pyrazinamide, and ethambutol for two months followed by rifampicin and ethambutol for seven months

B Start rifampicin, pyridoxine, and ethambutol for two months followed by rifampicin and pyridoxine for seven months

C Start rifampicin, pyridoxine, and pyrazinamide for two months followed by rifampicin and pyridoxine for four months

D Start rifampicin, pyridoxine, and pyrazinamide for four months followed by rifampicin and pyridoxine for four months

E Start rifampicin, pyridoxine, and pyrazinamide for six months followed by rifampicin and pyridoxine for four months

5. A 72-year-old male patient has been in ICU for five days. He is sedated and ventilated on a F$_i$O$_2$ of 0.75 and is receiving vaso-active support, haemodiafiltration, and total parenteral nutrition (TPN). He has a diagnosis of multiorgan failure secondary to acute severe gall-stone pancreatitis. Twelve hours earlier he had undergone a laparotomy to relieve abdominal compartment syndrome and has a laparostomy. He has not had any pancreatic tissue resected but intra-abdominal fluid was sent for culture. On returning from theatre, his oxygen requirements had increased from 0.45 to 0.75. You have been asked to review the patient as the nursing staff are concerned that his latest blood tests, taken 4 hours ago, show an increased white blood count (WBC) of 18 (from 14) and a C-reactive protein (CRP) of 285 (from 216). He also has a new low-grade pyrexia of 37.9°C and they are concerned re-garding his increased oxygen requirement. He is not on any antimicrobial agents but did receive prophylactic antibiotics intravenously consisting of cefuroxime 1.5 g and metronidazole 500 mg. During his time in theatre, his TPN line was disconnected.

The next most appropriate course of action is:

A Commence antibiotics for a ventilator-associated pneumonia

B Continue the prophylactic antibiotics already given intraoperatively (cefuroxime and metronidazole) until the results of microbiological culture of peritoneal fluid are known

C Start intravenous meropenem 1 g TDS as this patient is likely to have infected pancreatic necrosis

D Take blood cultures and commence vancomycin for suspected TPN line sepsis

E Take cultures for a full septic screen

6. A previously well five-month-old boy has been transferred to ICU from the paediatric ward following admission with a reduced level of consciousness. Earlier he had been refusing to feed and had loose bowel motions. At times his body feels stiff. He does not have a rash. A clinical diagnosis of possible bacterial meningitis has been made. Blood results are still awaited and a lumbar puncture has not yet been per-formed. No radiological imaging has been undertaken.

The next most appropriate course of action is:

A Administer IV amoxicillin

B Administer IV cefotaxime and ampicillin

C Administer IV ceftriaxone

D Administer IV ceftriaxone and vancomycin

E Perform a lumbar puncture and then give IV ceftriaxone

7. An 83-year-old man is in ICU recovering from an emergency laparotomy and subtotal colectomy performed for toxic megacolon secondary to *C. difficile* colitis. He had recently received antibiotic therapy.

Which of the following classes of antimicrobial agents is least likely to have caused his *C. difficile* colitis:

A Cephalosporins

B Lincosamides

C Penicillins

D Quinolones

E Tetracyclines

ANSWERS

Multiple-Choice Questions

1. TFFTF

Amphotericin is a mixture of two polyene macrolides (Amphotericin A and B) produced by *Streptomyces nodosus*. It is a fungistatic antibiotic which is active against a wide range of yeasts and yeast-like fungi including, but not solely limited to *Candida albicans*. The drug binds to cell membrane sterols, leading to altered membrane permeability and ultimately leakage of intracellular components. Ribosomal binding and subsequent protein inhibitions are a feature of tetracycline *antibacterial* agents. Deterioration of renal function may occur in up to 80% of patients who receive the drug. Amphotericin is poorly absorbed from the GI tract, which is why it may be used for selective oral decontamination of the gut.

Further reading

Scarth E, Smith S. *Drugs in Anaesthesia and Intensive Care*, 5th edition. Oxford University Press, 2016. Amphotericin.

2. FFFFF

Oseltamivir is a synthetic ethyl ester which is used in the treatment of influenza virus infections. It is an antiviral agent, which in its active form (oseltamivir carboxylate) selectively inhibits influenza A and B neuraminidase. At least 75% of an administered oral dose reaches the systemic circulation, but this is as *oseltamivir carboxylate*. Oseltamivir is a pro-drug and requires ester hydrolysis to convert it to its active form. Only 3% of the drug is protein bound in the plasma. Resistance mutations are usually viral subtype-specific and may be naturally occurring (i.e. no prior drug exposure is required).

Further reading

Scarth E, Smith S. *Drugs in Anaesthesia and Intensive Care*, 5th edition. Oxford University Press, 2016. Oseltamivir.

3. TFTTT

Fluorinated quinolones are derived from nalidixic acid. The mode of action of these drugs is to inhibit bacterial DNA gyrase, topoisomerase IV, and type II topoisomerases, thereby inhibiting bacterial DNA replication. Ciprofloxacin (one of several fluoroquinolones) can be used as a single agent against *Yersinia pestis* (plague) and may also be used for PEP against a number of bacterial bioterrorism organisms. Tendon rupture (Achilles) has been reported, a risk factor is co-administration of corticosteroids. Abdominal pain, nausea, vomiting, and neuropsychiatric disturbances have also been associated side effects of these drugs.

Further reading

Scarth E, Smith S. *Drugs in Anaesthesia and Intensive Care*, 5th edition. Oxford University Press, 2016. Fluoroquinolones.

4. FFFTF

Caspofungin is a semi-synthetic lipopeptide (echinocandin) compound synthesized from a fermentation product of *Glarea lozoyensis*. It has poor oral bioavailability. The drug inhibits *fungal* beta (1,3)-D-glucan. Beta (1,3)-D-glucan is not present in mammalian cells. It is highly protein bound (97% bound to albumin) but is not an inhibitor of cytochrome P450. It achieves fungicidal activity with lysis and death of hyphal apical tips and branch points where cell growth and division occur. It may be useful in treating isolates with acquired or intrinsic resistance to other agents (e.g. fluconazole, amphotericin B).

Further reading

Scarth E, Smith S. *Drugs in Anaesthesia and Intensive Care*, 5th edition. Oxford University Press, 2016. Caspofungin.

5. FFTFT

Aciclovir is an antiviral agent active against herpes simplex (I and II) and varicella-zoster virus. It is activated within the viral cell via phosphorylation by a virus-encoded thymidine kinase and thus has low toxicity for normal cells. Aciclovir triphosphate inhibits *viral* deoxyribonucleic acid (DNA) polymerase, which prevents further elongation of the viral DNA chain. Sars-CoV-2 is a ribonucleic acid (RNA) virus. The drug is eliminated by active tubular secretion in the urine (45–80% unchanged). Precipitation of the drug can occur in renal tubules if administered too rapidly or if the patient is poorly hydrated. Doses should be reduced in the context of renal impairment, and it is 60% removed by haemodialysis.

Further reading

Scarth E, Smith S. *Drugs in Anaesthesia and Intensive Care*, 5th edition. Oxford University Press, 2016. Aciclovir.

6. FFFTT

Carbapenems are beta-lactam derivatives and bind to penicillin-binding proteins on the bacterial cytoplasmic cell membrane, thereby blocking peptidoglycan synthesis and thus cell wall formation. Imipenem exhibits 20% plasma protein binding, meropenem exhibits 2% binding, and 85–95% for ertapenem. These drugs are broad-spectrum antibiotics, including activity against anaerobic bacteria. Seizure activity may occur by one of two mechanisms. Firstly, co-administration of imipenem and ganciclovir may lead to focal seizures. Carbapenems may also reduce sodium valproate levels, leading to seizure activity.

Further reading

Scarth E, Smith S. *Drugs in Anaesthesia and Intensive Care*, 5th edition. Oxford University Press, 2016. Carbapenems.

7. FFFFF

Neomycin, one of several aminoglycosides, is available in tablet form as a bowel sterilizing agent and to prevent hepatic coma. It is also available as a topical cream (bacterial skin infection and otitis externa) and an oral solution. Aminoglycoside drugs are active against Gram-positive and Gram-negative bacteria but not anaerobic organisms. They bind *irreversibly* to the bacterial 30S subunit of ribosomal proteins. They *prolong* the action of non-depolarizing muscle relaxants by inhibiting presynaptic acetylcholine release and stabilizing the post-synaptic membrane at the neuromuscular junction. These agents should be used with caution in patients with myasthenia gravis due to their effects on neuromuscular transmission, which could precipitate a myasthenic crisis.

Further reading

Scarth E, Smith S. *Drugs in Anaesthesia and Intensive Care*, 5th edition. Oxford University Press, 2016. Aminoglycosides.

Single Best Answers

1. C

This patient has neutropenic sepsis as evidenced by a neutrophil count of less than 0.5 × 10⁹ per litre together with a temperature of greater than 38°C. Suspected neutropenic sepsis should be considered an acute medical emergency and an immediate clinical assessment should be performed including a history and examination, together with blood tests which should include (but not limited to) a full blood count, C-reactive protein, lactate, and blood culture, including culture from any central venous access device if feasible (in this case, blood culture from the PICC line). While line infection might be the cause of this patient's infection, at this stage it is by no means certain and removal of the line would be premature without definitive evidence of infection. An opportunistic skin commensal organism may indeed be responsible for this infection (given the clinical signs of a skin infection on examination). However, at this stage of treatment it is too early to offer a limited antibacterial agent. Additional G-CSF doses have no part in the immediate management of neutropenic sepsis even if the patient is already receiving it. In addition, superadded doses of prophylactic antibiotics are not indicated in this scenario. NICE guidance states that all patients with suspected neutropenic sepsis should be offered beta-lactam monotherapy with piperacillin and tazobactam as initial empiric antibiotic therapy with or without an aminoglycoside unless there are patient-specific or local microbiological indications. Answer C is therefore the single best answer.

Further reading

NICE. Neutropenic Sepsis: Prevention and Management in People with Cancer, September 2012. Available at: https://www.nice.org.uk/guidance/cg151

Scarth E, Smith S. *Drugs in Anaesthesia and Intensive Care*, 5th edition. Oxford University Press, 2016. Aminoglycosides, Piperacillin.

2. E

This patient has high-severity community-acquired pneumonia based on CURB-65 scoring and as such has more than a 15% mortality risk. He should be treated with dual antibiotics comprised of a macrolide and in severe cases a beta-lactamase stable beta-lactam for seven to ten days, together with consideration for intensive care assessment and management.

Further reading

NICE. Pneumonia in Adults: Diagnosis and Management, December 2014. Available at: https://www.nice.org.uk/guidance/cg191/chapter/recommendations#hospital-acquired-pneumonia

Scarth E, Smith S. *Drugs in Anaesthesia and Intensive Care*, 5th edition. Oxford University Press, 2016. Macrolides, Penicillin.

3. E

Despite a viral aetiology being a possible precipitant for viral myocarditis, there is no evidence to support that administration of any antiviral agent in the acute setting affects outcome. The management of these patients is based on the best supportive care. There may be a role for individuals who have a chronic bacterial load several months after their initial presentation.

Further reading

Scarth E, Smith S. *Drugs in Anaesthesia and Intensive Care*, 5th edition. Oxford University Press, 2016. Oseltamivir.

4. A

This lady is at risk of multidrug-resistant TB given her history of working in areas with a prevalence of multidrug-resistant TB, likely exposure to cases of known multidrug-resistant TB and exposure to subtherapeutic doses of TB drug treatment. Absence of a BCG scar increases the risk of TB acquisition generally. Resistance to a single anti-TB agent requires modification of anti-TB therapy. In this case, answer A is the correct response.

Further reading

NICE. Tuberculosis, May 2016. Available at: https://www.nice.org.uk/guidance/ng33/chapter/recommendations#strategic-oversight-and-commissioning-of-tb-prevention-and-control-activities

5. E

Around 80% of deaths in patients with severe acute pancreatitis are related to infectious complications. There is no evidence for prophylactic antibiotics. While IV-line sepsis is a possibility, this should be confirmed before starting antibiotics. All ventilated patients are at risk of ventilator-associated pneumonia (VAP). But it is not unusual for an unwell ICU patient to have increased oxygen requirements following a laparotomy. Clear evidence of a VAP would then indicate appropriate antimicrobial therapy. Infected pancreatic necrosis should be considered in patients with pancreatic or extrapancreatic necrosis who deteriorate or fail to improve after seven to ten days, in which meropenem should be considered. A full septic screen and awaiting culture results is the best option.

Further reading

NICE. Pancreatitis, September 2018. Available at: https://www.nice.org.uk/guidance/ng104/chapter/Recommendations#acute-pancreatitis

Scarth E, Smith S. *Drugs in Anaesthesia and Intensive Care*, 5th edition. Oxford University Press, 2016. Cephalosporins, Metronidazole.

6. C

A lumbar puncture would be a high-risk procedure in a patient with a reduced level of consciousness (a possible sign of raised intracranial pressure). In addition, a lumbar puncture should not delay the administration of IV antibiotics. IV ceftriaxone with vancomycin is indicated in children and young people who have suspected bacterial meningitis and have had prolonged or multiple exposures to antibiotics. IV cefotaxime and ampicillin are used in children less than three months of age (due to the risk of Gram-negative bacilli infection or *Listeria monocytogenes* infection). IV amoxicillin is used in *confirmed* cases of *L monocytogenes* meningitis. IV ceftriaxone should be administered without delay in children aged three months or older with suspected bacterial meningitis.

Further reading

NICE. Meningitis (Bacterial) and Meningococcal Septicaemia in Under 16s: Recognition, Diagnosis and Management, February 2015. Available at: https://www.nice.org.uk/guidance/CG102/chapter/1-Guidance#management-in-secondary-care

Scarth E, Smith S. *Drugs in Anaesthesia and Intensive Care*, 5th edition. Oxford University Press, 2016. Cephalosporins, Penicillin.

7. E

C. difficile infection is associated with the use of broad-spectrum antibiotics. A NICE (National Institute for Health and Care Excellence) evidence summary demonstrated that tetracycline antibiotics had no significant association with *C. difficile* infection. Penicillins had an odds ratio of 2.71 to 3.25 with *C. difficile* infection. Quinolones had an odds ratio of

1.66 to 5.65. Clindamycin (which is a lincosamide antibiotic) had an odds ratio of 2.86 to 20.43. Cephalosporins had an odds ratio of 1.97 to 4.47.

Further reading

NICE. Clostridium Difficile Infection: Risk with Broad-Spectrum Antibiotics, March 2015. Available at: https://www.nice.org.uk/adv ice/esmpb1/chapter/Key-points-from-the-evidence

Scarth E, Smith S. *Drugs in Anaesthesia and Intensive Care*, 5th edition. Oxford University Press, 2016. Cephalosporins, Fluoroquinolones, Penicillin.

Intravenous fluids and blood products

Multiple-Choice Questions

1. Body fluid compartments:

A Due to its highly polar nature, water will distribute between all compartments

B Interstitial fluid has a similar electrolyte composition to plasma

C Intracellular fluid has a high sodium concentration and low potassium concentration

D Total body water makes up approximately 60% of total body weight

E Water is equally distributed between intracellular and intravascular compartments

2. Regarding human albumin solution (HAS)

A Albumin is the largest component of colloid oncotic pressure in blood

B Is a clear, straw-coloured fluid

C Is contra-indicated in immunocompromised recipients

D May prolong the action of warfarin

E The incidence of anaphylaxis is less compared to synthetic colloids

3. Regarding platelets

A All requested platelets will routinely be leucodepleted

B Group ABO-matched platelets are necessary for transfusion

C Have a shelf life of up to two months

D One adult dose of platelets may be from several donors

E Platelet components must not be placed in a refrigerator

4. Regarding fresh frozen plasma (FFP)

A Cryoprecipitate is formed from FFP

B FFP is first-line treatment for the reversal of warfarin

C Freezing is necessary to prevent bacterial growth

D It is not necessary to be group ABO specific for transfusion

E Must all be sourced from outside of the UK

5. Red blood cells

A A unit contains no clotting factors

B Have a shelf life of five days

C Leucodepletion is to reduce cytomegalovirus (CMV) risk

D Must be stored between 1–3°C

E Must not be warmed

6. Regarding sodium chloride

A 0.9% sodium chloride contains 154 milli-osmoles per litre

B 0.9% sodium chloride is isotonic with extracellular fluid

C Can cause a hyperchloraemic metabolic alkalosis

D Is completely absorbed when administered orally

E Normal saline contains buffering salts

7. Regarding Hartmann's solution

A Infusions of Hartmann's solution will not contribute to the development of acidosis

B Lactate is metabolized in all body cells

C Lactate is oxidized to glycogen and bicarbonate

D Lactate metabolism is increased by hypoxia

E Should not be administered with blood products

Single Best Answers

1. You have been called to the emergency department (ED) by the paediatric registrar. They have asked for assistance regarding the immediate treatment of a 2-week-old baby who has been brought into ED following diarrhoea and vomiting at home. You are shown two different intravenous (IV) fluids: 5% glucose and 0.9% normal saline. Comparing these two IV fluids, which of the following is most likely to be correct?

A 5% glucose is the resuscitation fluid of choice in neonates

B Both IV agents are effective volume expanders

C Both IV agents have equal osmolarity

D Dextrose is an isomer of glucose that cannot be metabolized

E The majority of glucose will move intracellularly

2. You are called urgently to the obstetric unit to assist with the management of a massive obstetric haemorrhage. As part of your immediate fluid resuscitation strategy, you are handed a 1 L bag of IV dextran. Considering the use of IV dextran, which of the following is most likely to be correct in the clinical context of massive obstetric haemorrhage?

A Can carry a blood-borne infection risk

B Dextrans are formed via the binding of two dextrose molecules

C Dextrans are recognized precipitants in thromboembolism

D Dextrans are unable to be renally excreted

E Do not interfere with cross-matching

3. You are assisting in the anaesthetic of a polytrauma patient who has sustained intra-thoracic, intra-abdominal, and pelvic blunt force trauma. A preoperative CT scan demonstrates the following injuries: right-sided pulmonary contusion with a flail segment; hepatic lacerations with associated haematoma formation; splenic rupture; free intra-abdominal fluid; and an undisplaced fracture of the right acetabulum. Regarding the use of red blood cell (RBC) transfusion in this patient, which of the following is most likely to be correct?

A During RBC storage there is no active cell metabolism

B Haematocrit of packed RBCs transfused is equivocal to whole blood haematocrit

C Large RBC transfusions can lead to hypercalcaemia

D The main degradation product of haemoglobin from RBC transfusion is bilirubin

E The main role of the RBC additive citrate is as a buffer

4. You have been asked to review a patient with longstanding chronic kidney disease. They have been admitted following an acute deterioration in their renal function secondary to diarrhoea and vomiting. Blood test results show an acute kidney injury 3 and severe metabolic acidosis. Treatments instigated so far include volume resuscitation, insertion of a urinary catheter, and medical treatment of hyperkalaemia. The patient is due to be transferred to the regional haemodialysis unit. Prior to patient transfer, the renal team have asked for the patient to receive sodium bicarbonate. Regarding the use of sodium bicarbonate, which of the following is most likely to be correct?

A 1.26% solution is hypertonic compared with plasma

B Can cause skin necrosis

C Can enhance the secretion of weak bases

D Is not absorbed through the gastrointestinal (GI) tract

E Will increase the potency of local anaesthetics

5. You have been called urgently to the endoscopy suite, where a patient is undergoing an oesophagoduodenoscopy (OGD) for bleeding oesophageal varices. A Sengstaken–Blakemore tube is being prepared to be inserted to gain haemostatic control. Your assistant is preparing a rapid infusion system, and a gelatin-type intravenous fluid is the priming agent. Regarding the use of gelatin-type fluids, which is the most appropriate answer?

A Due to the high incidence of anaphylaxis some agents are no longer commercially available

B Exert their effects through influencing capillary hydrostatic pressure

C Gelatins are animal collagen derivatives

D Have active metabolites

E May cause a type 1 von Willebrand-like syndrome

6. You are on the intensive care unit (ICU) ward round. A number of patients have been prescribed different IV fluids/blood products to be administered during the day. Which of the following is most accurate regarding the distribution of the following IV fluids/blood products?

A 20% HAS is initially distributed into the plasma and later equilibrates with the extracellular fluid

B Duration of fluid administration has no impact on distribution

C Hartmann's solution is initially distributed into the plasma and later equilibrates with the extracellular fluid

D Normal saline is initially distributed into the plasma and later equilibrates with all fluid compartments

E Packed red cells are initially distributed into the plasma and later equilibrates with the extracellular fluid.

7. You are preparing a teaching session for foundation doctors about the use of different IV fluids that they may be required to prescribe. Regarding the following IV fluids, which is the most appropriate answer?

A 5% glucose is isotonic with plasma

B 10% Glucose should only be administered via a central line

C Colloids consist of a base solution of sterile water with added synthetic proteins

D Hartmann's contains an equal proportion of calcium, potassium, and magnesium

E Ringer's acetate contains an equal proportion of calcium, potassium, and magnesium

ANSWERS

Multiple-Choice Questions

1. FTFTF

Water carries no charge and will therefore distribute evenly between compartments. Interstitial fluid has a similar electrolyte composition to plasma with a high sodium and low potassium concentration. Intracellular fluid has a low sodium concentration and high potassium concentration; potassium is actively transported into cells to maintain this gradient. Water is the largest component of the human body, averaging 60% of overall body weight. This figure will vary slightly according to age and body habitus. The main fluid compartments within the body can be defined as intracellular and extracellular. Extracellular fluid can be further split into intravascular fluid, transcellular fluid, and interstitial fluid. Two-thirds of body water is intracellular and one-third extracellular. Approximately 80% of extracellular fluid is interstitial, 20% intravascular, and a very small proportion is transcellular.

Further reading

Peck T, Hill S, Williams M. *Pharmacology for Anaesthesia and Intensive Care*, 4th edition. Cambridge University Press, 2014. Body fluid compartments pp. 286–287.

2. TTFFT

Albumin comprises the largest component of colloid oncotic pressure in the blood. HAS is a clear, straw-coloured fluid for infusion containing albumin of different concentrations, which has been pooled from the venous plasma of healthy subjects. It is a colloid used for plasma volume replacement in haemorrhage, burns, and in the treatment of hypoalbuminaemic states. As HAS is prepared from donor blood, there is a theoretical risk of blood-borne infections. It is, however, not contraindicated for use in immunocompromised individuals. Acidic drugs, such as warfarin, bind to albumin. Reductions in albumin concentration can therefore exaggerate the effects of such drugs. HAS, therefore, does not prolong the action of warfarin. Allergic reactions occur less frequently compared with synthetic colloids.

Further reading

Smith S, Scarth E. *Drugs in Anaesthesia and Intensive Care*, 5th edition. Oxford University Press, 2016. Human albumin solution.

3. TFFTT

All platelets have been leucodepleted at source since 1999. Group ABO-matched platelets are preferred but not essential for transfusion.

However, group O platelets should not be given to group A, B, or AB recipients unless they have been tested negative for high titre antibodies due to haemolysis risk. Pooled platelets suspended in platelet additive solution (PAS) have the plasma extracted and will also reduce the haemolysis risk. Platelets can be stored for up to five days between 20–24°C. An adult therapeutic dose (ATD) of platelets is obtained from the centrifugation of whole blood from four donations. A platelet-rich layer forms, which is pooled and re-suspended to create one unit. Alternatively, platelets can be obtained by single-donor apheresis. Platelet components must not be frozen or placed in a refrigerator.

Further reading

Provan D, Baglin T, Dokal I, De Vos J. *Oxford Handbook of Haematology*, 4th edition. Oxford University Press, 2014. Platelet transfusion pp. 768–769.

4. TFFTF

Cryoprecipitate is produced from FFP by slowly thawing it overnight, enabling cryoproteins (FVIII, von Willebrand factor (VWF), FXIII, fibronectin, and fibrinogen) to precipitate out of solution. Prothrombin complex concentrate and not FFP is recommended for the reversal of warfarin anticoagulation. FFP is obtained from whole blood donations or by apheresis. The reason plasma is rapidly frozen to less than –25°C is to maintain the activity of labile coagulation factors, rather than bacterial growth prevention. ABO-compatible FFP should be used as the first choice but is not mandatory. Group O FFP should only be given to group O patients, since it may contain a high titre of anti-A and anti-B antibodies. Donation units of FFP sourced from outside the UK are only indicated for all children born after 1996 to reduce the risk of transmission of vCJD.

Further reading

Provan D, Baglin T, Dokal I, De Vos J. *Oxford Handbook of Haematology*, 4th edition. Oxford University Press, 2014. Fresh frozen plasma pp. 770–771.

5. TFTFF

Units of RBCs do not contain any clotting factors. Units in the UK are supplied in an 'optimal additive solution' which allows the removal of all the plasma components and results in a less viscous product. Red blood cells have a shelf life of 35 days stored at 4°C. They should be stored between 2–6°C. All supplied blood in the UK has been leucodepleted at source since 1999; this provides adequate CMV risk reduction for the majority of situations. Specific CMV seronegative blood products should be used for intrauterine transfusions and neonates. Red blood cell packs may be warmed through appropriate fluid-warming devices, the transfusion should be given within 30 minutes of leaving the blood bank fridge.

Further reading

Provan D, Baglin T, Dokal I, De Vos J. *Oxford Handbook of Haematology*, 4th edition. Oxford University Press, 2014. Transfusion of red blood cells pp. 764–766.

6. FTFTF

Sodium chloride is a clear, colourless fluid available in a range of concentrations. 0.9% solution contains 154 mmol of sodium and 154 mmol of chloride per litre, its overall osmolality is 308 milli-osmoles per litre. 0.9% solution is isotonic with extracellular fluid and distributed uniformly throughout this compartment. Due to this high chloride content, it can promote hyperchloraemic acidosis, not alkalosis. It is rapidly and entirely absorbed when given orally. It contains no buffering salts, preservatives, or antimicrobial agents.

Further reading

Smith S, Scarth E. *Drugs in Anaesthesia and Intensive Care*, 5th edition. Oxford University Press, 2016. Sodium chloride.

7. FFTFT

Hartmann's solution is a crystalloid fluid with a similar electrolyte composition to plasma. Lactate is added to serve as an alternative source of bicarbonate; the main buffer component of the extracellular fluid. Infusions of Hartmann's solution may lead to respiratory acidosis as a result of carbon dioxide formed during lactate metabolism. Lactate is metabolized to glycogen, which is oxidatively metabolized to carbon dioxide and water. The carbon dioxide accepts an H+ ion to form bicarbonate. Conversion of lactate into bicarbonate and glycogen occurs only in the liver. This process is dependent on cellular oxidative activity which will be inhibited by liver dysfunction, acidosis, and hypoxic states. Hartmann's should not be administered with blood products as the calcium ions in the solution can lead to clotting of the blood product.

Further reading

Gupta A, Singh-Radcliff N. *Pharmacology in Anesthesia Practice*, 1st edition. Oxford University Press, 2013. Chapter 17.1 Crystalloids.

Smith S, Scarth E. *Drugs in Anaesthesia and Intensive Care*, 5th edition. Oxford University Press, 2016. Hartmann's solution.

Single Best Answers

1. E

Due to its limited effect on the intravascular volume, 5% glucose is not used as a resuscitation fluid for neonates. However, solutions containing a higher percentage of glucose are commonly used to treat neonatal hypoglycaemia. 5% glucose is not an effective volume expander.

Normal saline will distribute equally between the extracellular compartments, providing better volume expansion. Dextrose does refer to a dextro-rotatory isomer of glucose, but importantly it can be metabolized. The osmolarity of saline is 308 mOsm/L, compared with 278 mOsm/L of 5% glucose. Once infused into the intravascular space glucose is rapidly taken up into cells and metabolized, making E the correct answer. This gives an infusion of effectively free water, which is then equally distributed between all compartments; only a small portion is left intravascularly.

Further reading

Peck T, Hill S, Williams M. *Pharmacology for Anaesthesia and Intensive Care*, 4th edition. Cambridge University Press, 2014. Body fluid compartments pp. 286–287.

2. E

Dextrans do not interfere with cross-matching, making E the correct answer (although older preparations did). Dextrans are polysaccharide derivatives of sucrose, formed by the action of a bacterium containing the enzyme dextran sucrase. They are used for plasma volume replacement and in the prophylaxis of thromboembolism. Dextrans reduce ADP-induced platelet aggregation and decrease the effect of thrombin in platelets and thus exert an antithrombotic effect. Dextrans are available in different molecular weights, Dextran 40 and Dextran 70. Small molecules are excreted renally, and the large ones are metabolized by dextranases and excreted as carbon dioxide and water. Dextrans are synthetically produced and do not carry a blood-borne infection risk. The main side effect is severe hypersensitivity reactions, which occur in 1 in 3300 uses.

Further reading

Gupta A, Singh-Radcliff N. *Pharmacology in Anesthesia Practice*, 1st edition. Oxford University Press, 2013. Chapter 17.2 Colloids.

Smith S, Scarth E. *Drugs in Anaesthesia and Intensive Care*, 5th edition. Oxford University Press, 2016. Dextrans.

3. D

Bilirubin is the main product of haemoglobin degradation, increased levels may be detected when red blood cells are rapidly broken down, such as in haemolytic reactions. The haematocrit of packed red cells is much higher than whole blood, in the region of 70–80%. Large transfusions can lead to citrate toxicity, where citrate binds with calcium causing a hypocalcaemic state. This can cause cardiac depression and hypotension. Several products are added to red blood cells; citrate acts as an anticoagulant by binding calcium ions. Phosphate acts as a buffer and glucose provides an energy source. There is ongoing cell metabolism while in storage, hence the need for an energy source. Cooling helps slow this process.

Further reading

Gupta A, Singh-Radcliff N. *Pharmacology in Anesthesia Practice*, 1st edition. Oxford University Press, 2013. Chapter 17.3 Transfusion products.

Provan D, Baglin T, Dokal I, De Vos, J. *Oxford Handbook of Haematology*, 4th edition. Oxford University Press, 2014. Transfusion of red blood cells pp. 764–766.

4. B

1.26% sodium bicarbonate is almost isotonic with plasma, containing 150 mmol each of Na^+ and HCO_3- per litre, giving an osmolarity of 300 mOsm/L. It is highly irritant to tissues and may cause skin necrosis if extravasated. Sodium bicarbonate can be given orally and used as an antacid. It is water soluble and has a fast onset of action. It is absorbed through the GI tract, entering the systemic circulation and can cause metabolic alkalosis. Sodium bicarbonate will make the urine more alkaline and can enhance the secretion of weak acids, this may be utilized in aspirin overdose. The addition of sodium bicarbonate to local anaesthetics will raise the pH of the solution. This increases the unionized fraction of local anaesthetic available and thus increases the speed of onset time, not the potency.

Further reading

Peck T, Hill S, Williams M. *Pharmacology for Anaesthesia and Intensive Care*, 4th edition. Cambridge University Press, 2014. Bicarbonate pp. 290–291.

Smith S, Scarth E. *Drugs in Anaesthesia and Intensive Care*, 5th edition. Oxford University Press, 2016. Sodium bicarbonate.

5. C

Gelatins are a type of colloid fluid that can be used for plasma volume expansion. They are animal collagen derivatives produced by the thermal degradation of bovine gelatin. A significant side effect of gelatins is anaphylactic and anaphylactoid reactions, occurring in approximately 1 in 10,000 administrations. However, they remain available for use, products in the UK include Gelofusin® 4%, a succinylated gelatin, and Haemaccel® 3.5%, a urea-linked gelatin. They exert their effect by causing a temporary increase in plasma oncotic pressure, not hydrostatic pressure. Evidence regarding their effect on coagulation is inconclusive and they are not known to cause a type 1 von Willebrand-like syndrome. *In-vitro* studies suggest that gelatins are degraded by proteolytic enzymes into smaller peptides and amino acids. They do not have active metabolites.

Further reading

Peck T, Hill S, Williams M. *Pharmacology for Anaesthesia and Intensive Care*, 4th edition. Cambridge University Press, 2014. Gelatins pp. 287–289.

Smith S, Scarth E. *Drugs in Anaesthesia and Intensive Care*, 5th edition. Oxford University Press, 2016. Gelatins.

6. C

Multiple factors determine fluid distribution between body compartments, including the time over which the fluid is given. Other factors include the size and shape of molecules, hydrostatic pressure gradients, oncotic pressure gradients, and the endothelial barrier. Hartmann's and normal saline will initially be distributed into the plasma and due to the high sodium content with equilibrating within the extracellular space. 20% HAS remains within the plasma. It has a high oncotic pressure and will draw fluid into the intravascular space. Packed red cells will also remain within the plasma.

Further reading

Peck T, Hill S, Williams M. *Pharmacology for Anaesthesia and Intensive Care*, 4th edition. Cambridge University Press, 2014. Body fluid compartments pp. 286–287.

Smith S, Scarth E. *Drugs in Anaesthesia and Intensive Care*, 5th edition. Oxford University Press, 2016. Human albumin solution.

7. A

5% glucose has the same osmolality as plasma; it is isotonic. 5% glucose contains 278 mmol/L of glucose, with a matching osmolality of 278 mOsm/L. Hypertonic glucose solutions have a low pH and may cause venous irritation and thrombophlebitis, 20% or 50% glucose should be given via large central veins. Colloids are fluids which contain a base solution and electrolytes but with the addition of a colloid, a large molecule that does not diffuse across semi-permeable membranes. Colloids may be natural, for example albumin, or synthetic, such as gelatins and dextrans. Per litre, Hartmann's solution contains 2 mmol of calcium ions, 5 mmol of potassium ions, and no magnesium. Per litre, Ringer's acetate contains 1 mmol of calcium ions, 5 mmol of potassium ions, and 1 mmol of magnesium.

Further reading

Gupta A, Singh-Radcliff N. *Pharmacology in Anesthesia Practice*, 1st edition. Oxford University Press, 2013. Chapter 17.1 Crystalloids, Chapter 17.2 Colloids.

Smith S, Scarth E. *Drugs in Anaesthesia and Intensive Care*, 5th edition. Oxford University Press, 2016. Hartmann's solution.

Pharmacological principles

QUESTIONS

Multiple-Choice Questions

1. Regarding the removal of drug from the plasma in first-order kinetics

A Clearance is the amount of drug eliminated per minute

B The elimination rate of a given drug is constant

C The rate of elimination is equal to the clearance multiplied by the steady-state drug concentration

D Clearance by metabolic organs is proportional to its extraction ratio

E Flow limited drugs are those with an extraction ratio considerably less than 1

2. Regarding drug plasma concentration

A An intravenous loading dose is calculated by multiplying the desired plasma concentration by the drug's volume of distribution

B In steady-state conditions, the rate of drug elimination is in equilibrium with the rate of drug administration

C An oral maintenance dose is the hourly interval of administration multiplied by the elimination rate (per hour)

D During the terminal phase of elimination, a given drug's plasma concentration is equal to tissue concentrations

E An increasing bolus dose (e.g. of propofol) will increase the speed of onset of peak effect

3. Regarding elimination zero order kinetics

A The half-life is proportional to the drug concentration

B Clearance is a constant volume (l/kg) cleared of drug per unit of time

C Drug elimination rate is constant

D Concentration declines linearly over time

E Volume of distribution varies as plasma concentration varies at equilibrium

4. Consider a semilog plot depicting the log of drug concentration on the x-axis and the probability of analgesia on the y-axis

A A curve shifted to the left indicates greater potency

B Median effective dose (ED 50) describes drug efficacy

C A partial agonist will always have submaximal efficacy

D Efficacy is increased with increased drug affinity for its receptor (F)

E The effects of a competitive antagonist may be overcome with an increased dose of agonist

5. Bioavailability

A Is the fraction of the administered drug dose that undergoes first-pass metabolism

B An intravenously administered drug has 100% bioavailability

C Is calculated by dividing the area under the curve (AUC) of a plasma drug concentration vs. time plot after intravenous administration by the AUC after oral administration

D A drug administered completely via the sublingual route avoids first-pass metabolism

E First-pass metabolism, by definition, relates only to hepatic metabolism before the active drug reaches the systemic circulation

6. Regarding the metabolism of drugs

A Oxidative reactions include deamination

B Conjugation facilitates renal excretion through the removal of a polar group

C Is a major contributor to the terminal elimination phase of a drug

D Plasma clearance of suxamethonium is independent of hepatic blood flow

E Phase II biotransformation inactivates a drug

7. Concerning the excretion of drugs

A Biliary excretion is terminal elimination

B Increasing plasma protein binding decreases active tubular secretion

C An ionized weak acid or base is more rapidly excreted in the urine than a non-ionized drug

D The rate of excretion of a weak base may be increased by acidifying the urine

E The drug filtration rate is calculated by multiplying the glomerular filtration rate by the urinary drug concentration

Single Best Answers

1. A 62-year-old male is in the intensive care unit (ICU), having undergone an emergency Hartmann's procedure two days previously. He is sedated with propofol and remifentanil. A sedation break is planned with a view to possible tracheal extubation later that day. Which property of remifentanil best accounts for rapid weaning from sedation?

A 68% unionized at pH 7.4

B 70% plasma protein binding

C High potency

D Rapid ester hydrolysis

E Volume of distribution of 0.25–0.4 L/kg

2. A 20-year-old female is scheduled for incision and drainage of a perianal abscess. You plan total intravenous anaesthesia (TIVA) with target-controlled infusion (TCI) of propofol supplemented with alfentanil. Within the Marsh pharmacokinetic model, which element is of the most importance in determining the rate of infusion?

A Body mass index

B Concurrent opioid use

C Drug distribution

D Elimination half-life

E Infusion time

3. An 85-year-old female has arrived in theatre for management of a fractured neck of femur. A hemiarthroplasty is planned. Prior to spinal anaesthesia, you plan a femoral nerve block using a combination of lidocaine 1% with 1:200,000 adrenaline, and levobupivacaine 0.25%. What property of lidocaine is best attributable to its rapidity of onset of action?

A Lipid solubility

B Protein binding

C Site of administration

D Use of vasoconstrictor

E Volume of distribution

4. A 62-year-old male is undergoing an abdominoperineal resection. He is anaesthetised and ventilated with a mixture of desflurane, medical air, and oxygen. Which property of desflurane best accounts for its requirement of a Tec 6 vaporizer?

A Environmental toxicity

B High saturated vapour pressure

C Low blood:gas partition coefficient

D Low molecular weight

E Low oil:gas partition coefficient

5. An 80-year-old male patient is about to undergo an elective laparoscopic hernia repair. He has essential hypertension controlled by two antihypertensive agents. A total intravenous anaesthetic (TIVA) technique is chosen as part of his anaesthetic management. You are programming the TCI pump and are deciding which pharmacokinetic model to use. Which of the following would be the most appropriate to use?

A Use a plasma-target Marsh model

B Use a plasma-target Schneider model

C Use an effect-site Marsh model

D Use an effect-site Minto model

E Use an effect-site Schneider model

6. A 59-year-old male is listed for laparoscopic cholecystectomy. He has a body mass index (BMI) of 46, and a background of obstructive sleep apnoea. You plan TIVA with propofol and remifentanil. Which weight is the optimal choice in calculating a propofol dosage for induction of anaesthesia in the context of morbid obesity?

A 70 kg

B Actual body weight

C Adjusted body weight

D Ideal body weight

E Lean body weight

7. A patient with an eGFR >90 is receiving an infusion of drug 'Z' at a dose designed to maintain steady-state plasma concentration. The infusion is stopped after nine hours of administration and the context-sensitive half-time of the drug is measured at 300 minutes. Which drug is the patient most likely to have been receiving as drug 'Z'?

A Alfentanil

B Fentanyl

C Midazolam

D Propofol

E Thiopental

ANSWERS

Multiple-Choice Questions

1. FFTTF

Clearance is the volume of plasma from which a substance is removed per unit time. This may either be systemic clearance (including metabolism) or intercompartmental clearance. The elimination rate is the amount of drug eliminated per minute. Clearance is constant. The elimination rate varies on the given concentration within a volume, hence the need for clearance, which describes the constant volume of drug that is cleared in a given time. The rate of elimination is equal to the clearance multiplied by the steady-state drug concentration. Clearance by metabolic organs is proportional to its extraction ratio. Flow-limited drugs are those which are increasingly dependent on the blood flow to a given metabolic organ as the extraction ratio approaches 1. Capacity-limited drugs are those which are dependent on the metabolic activity of the organ, which would become impaired in liver impairment, for example.

Further reading

Freshwater-Turner D, Roberts F. Pharmacokinetics and anaesthesia. *BJA Education*, 2007;7(1):27–29.

O'Shaughnessy K. Principles of clinical pharmacology and drug therapy. In Warrell D, Cox T, Firth J (eds) *Oxford Textbook of Medicine*, Vol 1, 5th edition. Oxford University Press, 2010. Chapter 10.1.

2. TTFFF

When choosing a loading dose, the anaesthetist must consider the desired plasma concentration (c). A semilog plot may be used to help extrapolate the initial concentration of a drug upon administration (modelling for complete distribution (Vd [l/kg])). The dose is therefore a function of these two values (c.Vd). In steady-state conditions, the rate of drug elimination is in equilibrium with the rate of drug administration.

One may depict intermittent oral dosing: a drug is administered approximately every half-life to replenish the drug eliminated over that time. The same principle applies to constant infusions of a drug. However, the oral maintenance dose must also account for a fraction of oral bioavailability.

During the terminal phase of elimination, a given drug's plasma concentration is less than tissue concentrations. Drug returns from its distribution volumes to the plasma, where it undergoes permanent elimination.

Increasing a bolus dose will have no effect on the time of peak onset. It will increase the magnitude of such an effect, while the biophase remains constant.

Further reading

Freshwater-Turner D, Roberts F. Pharmacokinetics and anaesthesia. *BJA Education*, 2007;7(1):27–29.

O'Shaughnessy K. Principles of clinical pharmacology and drug therapy. In Warrell D, Cox T, Firth J (eds) *Oxford Textbook of Medicine*, Vol 1, 5th edition. Oxford University Press, 2010. Chapter 10.1.

3. TFTTF

The half-life is variable and is dependent on drug concentration.

The drug elimination rate is constant, often owing to the saturation of elimination processes. As the same amount of drug is eliminated per unit of time, a lesser concentration will achieve increased clearance. Clearance is therefore inversely proportional to the plasma concentration.

Concentration declines linearly over time. This is in contrast to first-order kinetics, in which the concentration declines logarithmically based on the half-life.

Regardless of zero-order kinetic elimination, the volume of distribution (Vd) remains constant as plasma concentration varies at equilibrium. Vd is dependent on the amount of drug present at a given time divided by the plasma concentration at that time.

Further reading

Freshwater-Turner D, Roberts F. Pharmacokinetics and anaesthesia. *BJA Education*, 2007;7(1):27–29.

O'Shaughnessy K. Principles of clinical pharmacology and drug therapy. In Warrell D, Cox T, Firth J (eds) *Oxford Textbook of Medicine*, Vol 1, 5th edition. Oxford University Press, 2010. Chapter 10.1.

4. TFTFT

A curve shifted to the left indicates that a lesser dose is required to produce a given clinical effect. This relates to greater drug potency.

As potency relates to the drug dosage required to produce a given clinical effect, the median effective dose (ED 50) is a standardized means of comparing drug potencies. It does not relate to drug efficacy, which describes the maximum of a given drug.

By definition, a partial agonist will always have submaximal efficacy. Clinically, however, a submaximal response may not always be evident.

Efficacy is independent of drug affinity for its receptor. It describes the maximal functional response of an already assumed drug-receptor complex. Potency is increased with increased receptor affinity.

While the effects of a competitive antagonist may be overcome with an increased dose of agonist, those of a non-competitive antagonist cannot.

Further reading

Freshwater-Turner D, Roberts F. Pharmacokinetics and anaesthesia. *BJA Education*, 2007;7(1):27–29.

Lambert D, McDonald J. Drug-receptor interactions in anaesthesia. *BJA Education*, 2022;22(1):20–25.

5. FTFTF

Bioavailability is the fraction of the administered drug dose that reaches systemic circulation in an active form.

By definition, an intravenously administered drug has 100% bioavailability.

Bioavailability is calculated by dividing the AUC of a plasma drug concentration vs. time plot after oral administration by the AUC after intravenous administration.

First-pass metabolism refers to drug metabolism following its 'first pass' through the liver following gastrointestinal absorption. Therefore, a drug administered completely via the sublingual route avoids first-pass metabolism.

Drugs can undergo enzymatic biotransformation in the gut wall. First-pass metabolism relates to both gut and hepatic metabolism before the active drug reaches the systemic circulation.

Further reading

Freshwater-Turner D, Roberts F. Pharmacokinetics and anaesthesia. *BJA Education*, 2007;7(1):27–29.

6. TFTTF

Amino acids undergo oxidative deamination. Other examples of oxidative metabolism include hydroxylation, dealkylation, and desulphurization.

Conjugation creates water-soluble molecules through the addition of a polar group, rendering it hydrophilic. This subsequently aids renal excretion.

Metabolism and excretion are the two determinants of the terminal elimination phase of a drug, during which the active drug is completely removed from the body.

Drugs such as remifentanil and suxamethonium are cleared by plasma and tissue ester hydrolysis. Their hepatic extraction ratio is therefore low, meaning their metabolism is independent of hepatic blood flow. In contrast, most anaesthetic drugs are cleared hepatically.

While most phase II biotransformed metabolites are inactive, some retain activity (e.g. metabolites of morphine and midazolam are as potent as the parent drug).

Further reading

Freshwater-Turner D, Roberts F. Pharmacokinetics and anaesthesia. *BJA Education*, 2007;7(1):27–29.

O'Shaughnessy K. Principles of clinical pharmacology and drug therapy. In Warrell D, Cox T, Firth J (eds) *Oxford Textbook of Medicine*, Vol 1, 5th edition. Oxford University Press, 2010. Chapter 10.1.

7. FFTTF

Metabolites excreted in the bile may undergo subsequent enterohepatic recycling, whereby it is reabsorbed into the circulation. Biotransformed metabolites may undergo hydrolytic reactions back to the parent drug.

Increasing plasma protein binding reduces glomerular filtration. It has no effect on active tubular secretion, which occurs while equilibrium is maintained between free drug and protein-bound drug.

Ionized weak acids and bases are more rapidly excreted in the urine than a non-ionized drug. Ionized drugs are polar. Their decreased lipid solubility leads to less passive reabsorption across renal tubular cells.

The rate of excretion of a weak base may be increased by acidifying the urine. The rate of excretion of a weak acid may be increased by alkalinizing the urine.

The drug filtration rate is calculated by multiplying the glomerular filtration rate by the free drug plasma concentration.

Further reading

O'Shaughnessy K. Principles of clinical pharmacology and drug therapy. In Warrell D, Cox T, Firth J (eds) *Oxford Textbook of Medicine*, Vol 1, 5th edition. Oxford University Press, 2010. Chapter 10.1.

Single Best Answers

1. D

Remifentanil has a context insensitive half time of 3–5 minutes. This facilitates rapid weaning in the context of a prolonged infusion. While all the aforementioned properties are true, of most relevance is the rapid hydrolysis by non-specific esterases within the plasma and tissues to a carboxylic acid derivative remifentanil acid. It is the quantity of these esterases that contribute to the drug's clearance of 4.2–5 L/min, which is independent of renal and hepatic function. This enzyme system cannot be saturated at even high concentrations of remifentanil.

Further reading

Smith S, Scarth E. *Drugs in Anaesthesia and Intensive Care*, 5th edition. Oxford University Press, 2016. Remifentanil.

2. D

A number of pharmocokinetic models for propofol exist including 'Marsh' and 'Schneider'.

Propofol administration should take into account lean body weight. Concurrent opioid use is important to consider with regard to desired effect-site concentration, as it will act synergistically with propofol. However, it does not form part of the Marsh pharmacokinetic model itself.

The distribution of propofol is based on a three-compartment pharmacokinetic model which is employed in TCI programmes.

Further reading

Absalom A, Mani V, De Smet T, Struys MM. Pharmacokinetic models for propofol—defining and illuminating the devil in the detail. *Br J Anaesth*, 2009;103(1):26–37.

Smith S, Scarth E. *Drugs in Anaesthesia and Intensive Care*, 5th edition. Oxford University Press, 2016. Propofol.

3. A

Lidocaine is 64–70% protein bound. A high degree of protein binding is associated with a long duration of action. pKa and lipid solubility are associated with a rapid onset time.

Its volume of distribution does not relate to the rapidity of onset.

Its site of administration, dose, and use of a vasoconstrictor influence its degree of systemic absorption. In order of decreasing absorption, sites include the intercostal, caudal, epidural, brachial plexus, and subcutaneous tissue.

Further reading

Smith S, Scarth E. *Drugs in Anaesthesia and Intensive Care*, 5th edition. Oxford University Press, 2016. Lidocaine.

4. B

In comparison to other inhalational anaesthetic agents, desflurane is noted to be the most environmentally toxic.

Due to its high saturated vapour pressure (SVP) at room temperature, a conventional vaporizer would require uneconomical levels of fresh gas flow to dilute it to clinically useful concentrations. This, in combination with a boiling point close to room temperature, and a resultant steep gradient in SVP with temperature change, necessitates a separate vaporizer.

Its low oil:gas partition coefficient and molecular weight relate to its potency and have no significant bearing on the type of vaporizer required. Its low blood:gas partition coefficient is related to a more rapid speed of onset in comparison to other inhalational anaesthetic agents.

Further reading

Smith S, Scarth E. *Drugs in Anaesthesia and Intensive Care*, 5th edition. Oxford University Press, 2016. Desflurane.

5. E

Using a Marsh pharmacokinetic model, either targeting a plasma or effect-site concentration will result in higher doses of propofol being administered to the patient both during induction and maintenance, compared with the use of the Schneider model targeting an effect-site concentration. This is due to the fact that the Schneider model modifies the induction and maintenance doses in relation to increasing age. Schneider does not target plasma concentration. Minto is a pharmacokinetic model used for remifentanil, not propofol.

Further reading

Absalom A, Mani V, De Smet T, Struys MM. Pharmacokinetic models for propofol—defining and illuminating the devil in the detail. *Br J Anaesth*, 2009;103(1):26–37.

Mulvey D, Al-Rifia Z. Principles of total intravenous anaesthesia: practical aspects of using total intravenous anaesthesia. *BJA Education*, 2016;16(8):276–280.

Smith S, Scarth E. *Drugs in Anaesthesia and Intensive Care*, 5th edition. Oxford University Press, 2016. Propofol.

6. E

In an obese patient, lean body weight is greater than ideal body weight.

In obesity, blood tends to distribute more towards non-adipose tissues. This may produce increased drug plasma concentrations if dosages are calculated as mg/kg based on actual body weight.

In morbidly obese patients, lean body weight should be used for TCI induction of anaesthesia. The total body weight should be used to calculate TCI maintenance.

Further reading

Mulvey D, Al-Rifia Z. Principles of total intravenous anaesthesia: practical aspects of using total intravenous anaesthesia. *BJA Education*, 2016;16(8):276–280.

Thompson J, Hebbes C. Pharmacokinetics of anaesthetic drugs at extremes of body weight. *BJA Education*, 2018;18(12):364–370.

7. B

Context-sensitive half-time (CSHT) is the time taken for the concentration of a drug to fall to 50% of its steady-state value following cessation of an infusion. Alfentanil, midazolam, propofol, and thiopental all have CSHTs, which increase as the duration of infusion increases until a plateau is reached. Out of these five drugs, fentanyl demonstrates the greatest magnitude of increase in CSHT—if plotted graphically, it would display a sigmoid-shaped curve.

Typical CSHT values following nine hours of infusion would be 80 mins for alfentanil, 80 mins for midazolam, 50 mins for propofol, and 200 mins for thiopental. Of interest remifentanil has a context-insensitive half-time, meaning its time to fall to 50% of its steady-state plasma concentration is independent of the duration of administration. This occurs because its metabolism is unsaturable due to the abundance of plasma and tissue esterases.

Further reading

Hill S. Pharmacokinetics of drug infusions. *Cont Educ Anaesth Crit Care Pain*, 2004;4(3):76–80.

Smith S, Scarth E. *Drugs in Anaesthesia and Intensive Care*, 5th edition. Oxford University Press, 2016. Remifentanil.

Drugs affecting the central nervous system

QUESTIONS

Multiple-Choice Questions

1. Regarding levetiracetam

A The mechanism of action of levetiracetam is through the blockade of voltage-gated sodium channels

B Levetiracetam is rapidly and almost completely absorbed orally with near 100% bioavailability

C It is completely hepatically metabolized to inactive metabolites

D Levetiracetam has a prolonged half-life of 36–42 hours

E The dose does not need to be reduced in renal impairment as it is metabolized in the liver

2. Regarding haloperidol

A It is a butyrophenone derivative

B The main mode of action is through dopaminergic agonism

C Its use may lead to dystonia and akathisia

D Can be used to treat hiccupping

E It should generally be administered intravenously due to its poor bioavailability

3. The following drugs are likely to cause induction of the cytochrome P450 system:

A Carbamazepine

B Gabapentin

C Levetiracetam

D Phenytoin

E Thiopental

4. The following are features of amitriptyline toxicity:

A Blurred vision

B Hypertension

C Hypersalivation

D Onset of clinical features within an hour of overdose

E Respiratory depression

5. The following drugs could be safely administered in a patient regularly taking phenelzine:

A Glycopyrrolate

B Metaraminol

C Phenylephrine

D Topical cocaine

E Tramadol

6. The following effects are likely to occur after intravenous administration of 1 g/kg mannitol:

A Reduced plasma viscosity

B Loss of cerebral autoregulation

C Reduced cerebral blood flow

D Increased renal blood flow

E Hypernatraemia

7. Regarding benzodiazepine toxicity:

A Features may include ataxia and nystagmus

B Propylene glycol poisoning should be considered

C Following oral administration, the peak effect is usually within 60–90 minutes

D May lead to rhabdomyolysis

E Treatment with flumazenil is recommended

Single Best Answers

1. You have an extremely anxious 30-year-old patient on your theatre list for surgical extraction of four wisdom teeth under general anaesthesia. She has a past medical history of generalized anxiety disorder and supraventricular tachycardia (for which she takes verapamil 40 mg TDS). Her body mass index is 18. Today is her second attendance to have this procedure. On the previous occasion, her anxiety increased to such an extent that she fled the admission ward in terror. She is desperate to have her surgical procedure and requests sedating oral premedication. When considering these various benzodiazepine drugs, which of the following statements is most accurate?

A Diazepam has poor oral bioavailability due to its poor lipid solubility

B Lorazepam has an intermediate duration of action due to strong γ-aminobutyric acid (GABA) receptor binding

C Midazolam has rapid action due to the opening of its imidazole ring at physiological pH

D Temazepam has low clearance, so it should be avoided in day surgery due to its prolonged duration of action

E The efficacy of midazolam is reduced by co-administration with verapamil

2. You are asked to review a patient on the intensive care unit. The patient is a 65-year-old female who is on day five of their admission following an emergency laparotomy for a perforated diverticulum, which resulted in four-quadrant faecal peritonitis. The patient was extubated two days ago, but is requiring ongoing vasopressor support for the treatment of her sepsis. She was noted to be agitated on that morning's consultant-led ward round and a plan was documented to prescribe dexmedetomidine if her agitation did not improve. Which is the most accurate description for this drug's sedative effects?

A Agonism at the locus coeruleus increasing potassium conductance

B α-adrenergic agonism to α2: α1 receptors in a ratio of 80:1

C Direct α2 agonism in the cortex

D GABA agonism, modulating noradrenaline release

E Hyperpolarization in the spinal cord dorsal horns

3. You are called to the emergency department (ED) to attend to a 25-year-old male with known poorly controlled epilepsy and severe autism. He has presented to the ED in status epilepticus—this is his fourth admission in the past 12 months. The ED registrar administers a rapid bolus of drug 'X' at an appropriate dose to the patient to attempt to control their seizures. Two minutes later you observe that the patient has become apnoeic and when you look at the electrocardiograph (ECG) trace on the patient's bedside monitor, you diagnose a complete heart block.

Which of the following drugs is most likely to be drug 'X'?

A Diazepam

B Levetiracetam

C Lorazepam

D Phenytoin

E Sodium valproate

4. You have an obese 45-year-old female patient on your theatre list, booked for an elective laparoscopic cholecystectomy following their acute presentation of gallstones six months previously. Her liver function tests and amylase were mildly deranged during her previous admission; however, they have returned to baseline now on her preassessment blood tests. Past medical history includes epilepsy, which is controlled with carbamazepine. She has not experienced a seizure for five years and holds a driving licence. She is anxious about the implications of anaesthesia. Regarding her carbamazepine, which of the following effects should you be most aware of when planning her anaesthetic?

A Administering metronidazole will reduce plasma carbamazepine concentrations

B It decreases minimum alveolar concentration (MAC) requirements

C It prolongs the duration of activity of aminosteroid neuromuscular blocking drugs

D It shortens the duration of action of therapeutic fentanyl

E Its use increases sensitivity to ephedrine

5. You are asked to anaesthetise a 33-year-old female patient with myasthenia gravis. Her weight is 72 kg. Daily medication includes pyridostigmine 60 mg qds, prednisolone 30 mg daily, and azathioprine 75 mg bd. The patient is listed for elective fixation of a large midline incisional hernia which has been becoming increasing tender recently and the surgeons are keen that her surgery is expedited. Which of the following would be most appropriate to use during her anaesthetic?

A Atracurium 35 mg

B Mivacurium 15 mg

C Rocuronium 15 mg

D Suxamethonium 75 mg

E Vecuronium 12 mg

6. You have been called to review a 47-year-old female patient in intensive care who has been treated for delirium with clonidine, midazolam, and haloperidol. They have become progressively more agitated and are observed to be sweating and blinking rapidly. When you examine them, you note their eyes have fixed deviation with upward and lateral gaze. They are also lacrimating and have a flushed facial appearance. You request the nurse to check the patient's temperature due to the sweating/flushing which she reports back as 36.9°C. The patient's pulse is elevated at 113 bpm.

Which drug treatment option would you consider the most appropriate management plan?

A Amisulpride

B Neostigmine/glycopyrronium bromide combination

C Olanzapine

D Prochlorperazine

E Procyclidine

7. You attend the ward to preassess a 69-year-old male patient listed on the trauma list for fixation of a hip fracture. The patient was admitted six hours ago, and the ward pharmacist is at the patient's bedside performing medicines reconciliation. They report to you that there is a drug not presently accounted for on the patient's ward drug chart that they note to be in the patient's multi-compartment compliance aid. The patient tells you they were prescribed this drug for the treatment of depression and recalls they initially experienced nausea and abdominal pain but this settled with time. They were also instructed by their GP not to stop this medication abruptly.

If you were given the following additional information, which drug would you consider this most likely to be:

- Drug mechanism specifically involves 5-hydroxytryptamine
- Metabolism is via hepatic cytochrome p450 system
- Known to inhibit cytochrome p450
- Side effects include hyponatraemia, altered taste, and increased risk of bleeding

A Amitriptyline

B Bupropion

C Duloxetine

D Isocarboxazid

E Sertraline

ANSWERS

Multiple-Choice Questions

1. FTFFF

Levetiracetam, is a pyrrolidone derivative with a different mechanism of action to the other antiepileptic agents available. It appears to bind to synaptic vesicle protein 2A, therefore inhibiting intraneuronal calcium release. It is rapidly and completely absorbed with extremely high bioavailability. It is minimally metabolized (24%) via hepatic hydrolysis to an inactive metabolite and renally eliminated. As a result, the dose should be reduced in patients with a glomerular filtration rate of less than 80 ml/min/1.73 m^2. Drug half-life is around seven hours. Administration is not associated with cognitive impairment or drug-induced weight gain but may cause behavioural changes and somnolence.

Further reading

Lyseng-Williamson KA. Levetiracetam: a review of its use in epilepsy. *Drugs*, 2011; 71(4):489–514.

Smith S, Scarth E. *Drugs in Anaesthesia and Intensive Care*, 5th edition. Oxford University Press, 2016. Levetiracetam.

2. TFTTF

Haloperidol is a butyrophenone derivative that is commonly used for the management of acute confusional states. In addition, it is a potent antiemetic owing to central dopaminergic (D_2) blockade. It also antagonizes post-synaptic GABA receptors and α-adrenergic receptors.

Dystonias are sustained muscle contractions causing repetitive abnormal movements. Akathisia is characterized by restlessness and appears to be a dose-related phenomenon. These may occur within a few hours of administration but sometimes take a number of days. These extrapyramidal side effects are relatively common with the use of haloperidol and can include neuroleptic malignant syndrome.

It is well absorbed orally with a bioavailability of 50–88%. It is highly protein bound with a large volume of distribution. Elimination depends on the route of administration but the half-life can be anywhere from 10 to 38 hours.

Further reading

Espi Forcen F, Matsoukas K, Alici Y. Anti-psychotic induced akathisia in delirium: a systematic review. *Palliat Support Care*, 2016;14(1): 77–84.

Smith S, Scarth E. *Drugs in Anaesthesia and Intensive Care*, 5th edition. Oxford University Press, 2016. Haloperidol.

3. TFFTT

Cytochrome P450 are a family of haem-containing enzymes, some of which are found in the liver and are essential for metabolism by oxidation to a more water-soluble form of a wide variety of medications. The isoform nomenclature is based on the similarities between amino acid sequences with families coded numerically, subfamilies alphabetically from A to E and specific genes then coded numerically. The CYP3A family metabolizes around 40–50% of known drugs. Enzyme induction takes place over several days or weeks.

Phenytoin, carbamazepine, and barbiturates are all inducers of the cytochrome P450 system, affecting a number of cytochrome enzymes including 1A2, 2C, and 3A4. Unlike many other antiepileptic agents, levetiracetam does not induce the CYP450 system. Gabapentin does not appear to affect the CYP450 system.

Some important anaesthetic substrates that may be affected by induction or inhibition of the CYP enzyme responsible for their metabolism include ketamine (CYP2B6); ibuprofen and diclofenac (CYP2C9); tramadol, codeine, oxycodone (CYP2D6); isoflurane and sevoflurane (CYP2E1); alfentanil, bupivacaine, midazolam, ondansetron, fentanyl (CYP3A4). Some drugs can be metabolized by a number of different enzymes; for instance, paracetamol (CYP1A2, CYP2E1, CYP3A4), lidocaine (CYP1A2, CYP3A4), and ropivacaine (CYP1A2, CYP3A4). Note that the likelihood of a clinically significant interaction will depend on a number of factors including oral bioavailability, the hepatic extraction ratio (i.e. whether drug metabolism is perfusion or enzyme limited) and the availability of alternative metabolic pathways.

Further reading

Asadi-Pooya AA, Sperling MR. *Antiepileptic Drugs: A Clinician's Manual*, 2nd edition. Oxford University Press, 2010. Clinically important drug interactions with antiepileptic drugs.

Hardman JG, Hopkins PM, Struys MMRF. *Oxford Textbook of Anaesthesia*. Oxford University Press, 2017. Drug interactions in anaesthetic practice.

Martin A, Scahill L, Kratochvil C. *Pediatric Psychopharmacology*, 2nd edition. Oxford University Press, 2010. Cytochrome P450-mediated drug interactions.

4. TFFFT

Clinical features of tricyclic antidepressant overdose are usually apparent within four hours of overdose. Anticholinergic effects are initially apparent including blurred vision, dryness of the mouth, constipation, urinary retention, and drowsiness. Toxicity may result in pyramidal signs, acidaemia, respiratory depression, and sedation. Decreasing pH increases the tricyclic antidepressant binding to sodium channels causing blockade resulting in QRS prolongation, arrhythmias (including ventricular tachycardia and fibrillation) and seizures. Hypotension results from α adrenoreceptor antagonism.

Management includes supportive measures and active correction of acidaemia.

Amitriptyline has an oral bioavailability of 45% and is highly protein bound with a large volume of distribution. Metabolism occurs by N-demethylation and hydroxylation with subsequent conjugation to glucuronide and sulphate. Nortriptyline is an intermediate active metabolite. The elimination half-life is 12.9–36.1 hours.

Tricyclic antidepressants remain a second-line therapy in depression, but are also used as an adjunct in chronic pain management. Other examples include dosulepin, imipramine, and nortriptyline. Their therapeutic effect is a result of inhibiting the presynaptic reuptake of noradrenaline and serotonin within the central nervous system (CNS). In addition, they antagonize muscarinic cholinergic, α-1 adrenergic, and H_1 and H_2 histaminergic receptors causing a wide range of side effects, which may include fatigue, sedation, and weakness.

Further reading

Bateman N, Jefferson R, Thomas S, Thompson J, Vale A. *Toxicology (Oxford Desk Reference)*. Oxford University Press, 2014. CNS Drugs.

Smith S, Scarth E. *Drugs in Anaesthesia and Intensive Care*, 5th edition. Oxford University Press, 2016. Amitriptyline.

5. TFTFF

Phenelzine is an antidepressant leading to the inhibition of monoamine oxidase (MAO) A and B through irreversible binding. Monoamine oxidase is an enzyme present on mitochondrial membranes. MAO-A preferentially metabolizes serotonin, noradrenaline, and adrenaline while MAO-B metabolizes non-polar aromatic amines. Moclobemide is a newer reversible MAO-A inhibitor, and of note, the antibiotic linezolid is a reversible non-selective monoamine oxidase inhibitor (MAOI).

Of greatest importance with regards to the MAOIs is the possibility of precipitating serotonin syndrome if drugs with serotonergic effects (such as pethidine and tramadol) are co-administered or of grossly exaggerated hypertensive effects from indirect sympathomimetics (such as metaraminol, ephedrine, and cocaine). In addition, MAOIs markedly exaggerate the depressant effect of volatiles on blood pressure and CNS and inhibit plasma cholinesterase, prolonging the duration of suxamethonium.

Direct sympathomimetics such as phenylephrine and adrenaline can be administered with caution. Anticholinergics such as glycopyrrolate can be safely used. Morphine can be used safely although MAOIs can inhibit hepatic microsomal enzymes, therefore prolonging the action of opioids and enhancing their effect. To avoid the potential perioperative complications, irreversible MAOIs may be discontinued for at least two weeks (to allow for the regeneration of new enzymes) before proceeding with elective surgery, but only after consultation with a psychiatrist. Moclobemide may be omitted for 24 hours preoperatively.

Further reading

Allman K, Wilson I, O'Donnell A. *Oxford Handbook of Anaesthesia*, 4th edition. Oxford University Press, 2015. Psychiatric disorders and drugs.

Smith S, Scarth E. *Drugs in Anaesthesia and Intensive Care*, 5th edition. Oxford University Press, 2016. Phenelzine.

6. TFFTF

Mannitol is a low-molecular-weight alcohol presented as a hyperosmolar fluid used to reduce the volume and therefore the pressure of cerebrospinal fluid (CSF). It decreases the rate of CSF formation and reduces brain extracellular water across the blood–brain barrier (which it does not cross when intact) into the plasma. The early plasma expansion reduces blood viscosity, which can aid regional cerebral microvascular flow and oxygenation.

It is freely filtered in the kidney and not reabsorbed, increasing the osmolality of the filtrate and may lead to a diuresis five times that of the administered volume.

Doses range from 0.25 to 1 g/kg with an action within a few minutes, lasting for 1–4 hours. Immediately after administration, it can be expected to increase blood pressure. It will lead to a significant reduction in intracranial pressure (ICP) with preservation of blood flow when autoregulation is intact. When autoregulation is defective it will lead to a minimal reduction in ICP with an increase in cerebral blood flow as vasoconstriction will not occur in response to reduced viscosity. Renal blood flow will also increase due to increased intravascular volume and the rate of renin secretion will fall. Diuresis of poorly concentrated urine will occur after 1–3 hours. Plasma sodium and potassium may fall with high doses.

Further reading

Nathanson M, Moppett IK, Wiles M. *Neuroanaesthesia (Oxford Specialist Handbooks in Anaesthesia)*. Oxford University Press, 2011. Pharmacology.

Smith S, Scarth E. *Drugs in Anaesthesia and Intensive Care*, 5th edition. Oxford University Press, 2016. Mannitol.

Wijdicks EFM, Clark SL. *Neurocritical Care Pharmacotherapy: A Clinician's Manual*. Oxford University Press, 2018. Osmotic therapy.

7. TTTTF

Benzodiazepines act via benzodiazepine receptors linked to $GABA_A$ receptors, enhancing the effect of GABA neurotransmitter, causing an increase in chloride permeability resulting in neuronal hyperpolarization, therefore decreasing excitability.

Peak effects after oral administration are typically within 60–90 minutes. The offset will depend on a number of factors including redistribution to fat and elimination. They are hepatically metabolized and so severe liver disease will delay elimination and increase the risk of toxicity. A number of benzodiazepines when metabolized will produce active compounds which can contribute to the toxic effects (diazepam in particular). Metabolites are renally excreted.

Features of overdose include drowsiness, ataxia, dysarthria, and nystagmus. Coma, hypotension, bradycardia, and respiratory depression can follow especially if taken in conjunction with alcohol or opioids. Hypothermia and rhabdomyolysis have occurred in severe cases.

Parenteral preparations of diazepam and lorazepam contain propylene glycol as a diluent. Prolonged administration, e.g. by continuous infusion, can rarely result in propylene glycol poisoning. Features can include severe lactic acidosis, cardiac arrhythmias, and skin necrosis. Of note, phenytoin also has propylene glycol as a diluent.

Although flumazenil is a competitive antagonist at benzodiazepine receptors and can therefore reverse the effects, it should be used with extreme caution as it may precipitate withdrawal or seizures. Its half-life is only 45–90 minutes, which is considerably less than the majority of benzodiazepines.

Further reading

Bateman N, Jefferson R, Thomas S, Thompson J, Vale A. *Toxicology (Oxford Desk Reference)*. Oxford University Press, 2014. CNS Drugs.

Nageshwaran S, Ledingham D, Wilson HC, Dickenson A. *Drugs in Neurology*. Oxford University Press, 2017. Benzodiazepines.

Wijdicks EFM, Clark SL. *Neurocritical Care Pharmacotherapy: A Clinician's Manual*. Oxford University Press, 2018. Antidotes with overdose.

Single Best Answers

1. B

Diazepam is well absorbed orally and is highly lipid soluble and so has a rapid onset but results in redistribution and can accumulate. It has active metabolites that prolong its duration of action. Lorazepam is poorly lipid-soluble resulting in a slower onset of action and a small V_D. It binds to GABA receptors strongly prolonging its effect. It does not form active metabolites. Midazolam owes its potency to high lipid solubility and receptor affinity. Its imidazole ring opens in acidic pH conferring water solubility. It comes prepared in a solution with a pH of 3.5. At physiological pH, the ring closes leading to lipid solubility thus rapid onset. Its high clearance, lipophilicity, and rapid elimination results in a short duration of action. Despite metabolites having minimal activity, renal failure may prolong the effects.

Temazepam has a relatively high clearance and small V_D and therefore has a relatively short duration of action. Benzodiazepines are formed from a benzene ring (5-carbon) joined to a diazepine ring (2-nitrogen,

5-carbon) with a variety of side groups accounting for the differences between drugs. The different properties of some common benzodiazepines are summarized in Table 10.1. Of note, higher lipid solubility is associated with a quicker onset. Elimination is through the hepatic p450 system and glucuronide conjugation. Indications for verapamil include the management of tachyarrhythmias, angina, and hypertension. Study evidence suggests an increased exposure to midazolam should be expected with co-administration and manufacturers advise dose adjustment.

Further reading

Gupta A, Singh-Radcliff N. *Pharmacology in Anesthesia Practice*. Oxford University Press, 2013. Benzodiazepines.

Nageshwaran S, Ledingham D, Wilson HC, Dickenson A. *Drugs in Neurology*. Oxford University Press, 2017. Benzodiazepines.

Smith S, Scarth E. *Drugs in Anaesthesia and Intensive Care*, 5th edition. Oxford University Press, 2016. Diazepam, Lorazepam, Midazolam, Temazepam.

2. A

Dexmedetomidine is an imidazole derivative producing sedation, anxiolysis, and analgesia that is increasingly used for sedation in critical care patients.

It is an α-adrenergic agonist to α2:α1 receptors in a ratio of 1600:1 although this selectivity decreases with rapid administration. Their activation leads to increased potassium conductance causing hyperpolarization in the locus coeruleus, reducing activity in the noradrenergic pathways associated with arousal and vigilance and increasing stage 3 non-rapid eye movement sleep (N3). Its analgesic effects are due to its action on α2 receptors in the dorsal horns. In contrast, other anaesthetic agents such as barbiturates act on inhibitory GABAergic interneurons.

It causes a predictable decrease in mean arterial pressure and heart rate with no clinically significant respiratory depression. It decreases plasma adrenaline and noradrenaline concentrations and blunts the sympathetic response to surgery. It may cause fever, nausea, and discontinuation may lead to withdrawal reactions.

It has a distribution half-life of six minutes and is highly protein bound with a V_D of 1.33 L/kg. It undergoes hepatic metabolism by glucuronidation and *N*-methylation. 95% is excreted in the urine with a clearance of 39 L/hr and the half-life is two hours. Of note, it crosses the placenta.

Further reading

Gupta A, Singh-Radcliff N. *Pharmacology in Anesthesia Practice*. Oxford University Press, 2013. Dexmedetomidine.

Pryor KO, Veselis RA. *Neuroscientific Foundations of Anesthesiology*. Oxford University Press, 2011. Anesthetic modulation of memory processing in the medial temporal lobe.

Table 10.1 Pharmacokinetic parameters of some common benzodiazepines

	Half-life (hrs)	Half-life of active metabolite (hrs)	Oral bioavailability (%)	Lipid solubility	Protein binding (%)	Volume of Distribution (l/kg)	Active metabolites	Clearance (ml/min/kg)
Midazolam	2–3	–	44	High	96	0.8–1.5	Minimal	5.8–9
Temazepam	5–11	–	100		76	0.8	Minimal	6.6
Lorazepam	8–25	–	90	Poor	88–92	1	None	1
Diazepam	20–40	100	86–100	High	99	0.8–1.4	Desmethyl-diazepam, oxazepam, temazepam	0.32–0.44

Smith S, Scarth E. *Drugs in Anaesthesia and Intensive Care*, 5th edition. Oxford University Press, 2016. Dexmedetomidine.

Stevens RD, Hart N, Herridge MS. *Textbook of Post-ICU Medicine: The Legacy of Critical Care*. Oxford University Press, 2014. Sleep disorders and recovery from critical illness.

3. D

Rapid boluses of phenytoin may result in hypotension, arrhythmias including complete heart block and ventricular fibrillation, and respiratory arrest. For this reason, when administered as a bolus, patients should be fully monitored, and the infusion slowed down or stopped should adverse features become apparent. The other agents mentioned are unlikely to result in arrhythmias in this situation, although benzodiazepines may result in respiratory arrest.

Phenytoin acts as a membrane stabilizer (rather than increasing the seizure threshold), by slowing inward sodium and calcium and outward potassium flux during depolarization in excitable tissue. As such it is a class I antiarrhythmic, shortening the cardiac action potential.

Oral absorption is 85–95% complete. It is highly protein bound with a small V_D. It is predominantly metabolized by CYP2C9. It is a potent enzyme inducer of CYP2C9, CYP2C19, CYP1A2, and CYP3A4. Due to autoinduction, the dose may need to be increased, but this process takes several days to weeks.

Phenytoin exhibits zero-order kinetics, otherwise known as nonlinear kinetics, just above the therapeutic range; a small increase in an administered dose produces a much larger increase in plasma level. Hypoalbuminaemia, uraemia, hepatic disease, foods, and drugs may all influence free (i.e. active) levels.

Further reading

Asadi-Pooya A, Sperling M. *Antiepileptic Drugs: A Clinician's Manual*, 2nd edition. Oxford University Press, 2015. Monitoring antiepileptic drugs and their toxicity.

Nageshwaran S, Ledingham D, Wilson HC, Dickenson A. *Drugs in Neurology*. Oxford University Press, 2017. Phenytoin and fosphenytoin.

NICE. Phenytoin, 2022. Available at: https://bnf.nice.org.uk/drug/phenytoin.html#sideEffects

Smith S, Scarth E. *Drugs in Anaesthesia and Intensive Care*, 5th edition. Oxford University Press, 2016. Phenytoin.

4. D

Carbamazepine is an iminostilbene derivative related to the tricyclic antidepressants. It is used in the management of epilepsy, bipolar disorder, and trigeminal neuralgia. It causes a use-dependent block of neuronal voltage-gated sodium channels and stabilizes neurons by inhibition at L-type calcium channels. It is only available as an oral formulation.

It has 100% oral bioavailability and is 75% protein bound with a V_D of 1 l/kg. It is hepatically metabolized to an active epoxide and is a CYP3A4 enzyme inducer. It is excreted unconjugated in the urine and has an elimination half-life of 16–36 hours, which reduces with enzyme autoinduction over a number of weeks. Aminosteroid efficacy is reduced in patients on long-term carbamazepine.

Long-term use of carbamazepine increases hepatic fentanyl clearance, which may result in decreased durations of therapeutic concentrations and hence patients may need higher or additional doses of fentanyl in order to obtain satisfactory pain relief. Carbamazepine does not increase sensitivity to sympathomimetic drugs and does not decrease MAC requirements. Common side effects include nausea, drowsiness, and ataxia. Co-administration with metronidazole risks inhibiting carbamazepine metabolism, leading to potentially toxic plasma concentrations.

Further reading

Nageshwaran S, Ledingham D, Wilson HC, Dickenson A. *Drugs in Neurology*. Oxford University Press, 2017. Carbamazepine and related antiepileptic drugs.

Nozari A, et al. Prolonged therapy with the anticonvulsant carbamazepine leads to increased plasma clearance of fentanyl. *J Pharm Pharmacol*, 2019;71(6):982–987.

Smith S, Scarth E. Drugs in Anaesthesia *and* Intensive Care, 5th edition. Oxford University Press, 2016. Carbamazepine.

5. C

Myasthenia gravis is an autoimmune condition where IgG antibodies form against the post-synaptic acetylcholine receptor. It is characterized by fatigable muscle weakness and frequently involves ocular symptoms.

Pyridostigmine is an acetylcholinesterase inhibitor. Acetylcholinesterase is the enzyme found at the neuromuscular junction responsible for the degradation of acetylcholine, breaking it down to acetate and choline. Acetylcholinesterase inhibitors act by reversibly binding to acetylcholinesterase preventing the breakdown of acetylcholine, therefore increasing the amount available to generate an action potential. In myasthenia gravis, pyridostigmine is used for its longer duration of action. In contrast, the duration of edrophonium and neostigmine is shorter; 10 minutes and 40–60 minutes with peak effects at 0.8–2 minutes and 7–11 minutes, respectively. Along with neostigmine and edrophonium, pyridostigmine does not cross the blood–brain barrier due to the presence of a quaternary ammonium group. Other drugs which may be utilized in the management of the condition include azathioprine and glucocorticoids for their immunosuppressive actions.

As a general principle, neuromuscular blocking drugs should be avoided in patients with myasthenia and achieving muscle relaxation via sufficient anaesthetic depth is preferable or the use of regional or local anaesthetic techniques if possible. Careful anaesthetic management is even more critical if patients are established on acetylcholinesterase inhibitor medications.

If the use of neuromuscular blocking drugs is unavoidable, then non-depolarizing agents should be used. Due to the unpredictable response and the decreased numbers of functional acetylcholine receptors in myasthenia gravis, small doses of such agents should be given with titration to effect guided by a train of four monitor. Receptor density is typically 30% of normal levels hence dose requirement is often approximately 30% of a standard intubating drug dose (NB: intubating doses are typically quoted as 0.6 mg/kg rocuronium; 0.5 mg/kg atracurium; 0.1 mg/kg vecuronium). Some sources however recommend even smaller initial doses such as 0.1–0.2 of the ED^{95} dose be used. Intubating doses are typically 2–3 × ED^{95} doses, so very small doses may need to be repeated.

Depolarizing agents such as suxamethonium should be avoided completely as patients are typically resistant to their effect and additionally pyridostigmine, due to its action on pseudocholinesterase, may reduce its metabolic destruction. Mivacurium is also metabolized by plasma pseudocholinesterase so its metabolism would be similarly inhibited. Sugammadex is recommended for reversal due to unpredictability when using an anticholinesterase agent (neostigmine), hence the selection of rocuronium or vecuronium may be considered preferential over atracurium as a blocking agent should reversal be required. The dose of vecuronium presented would be completely excessive. If suxamethonium was utilized, then due to the reduced receptor density approximately 2.6× normal dose would actually need to be selected—however, there would be a significant chance of phase II block occurring with this. Of note, azathioprine has been associated with prolongation of the effects of suxamethonium and inhibition of non-depolarizing muscle relaxant agents.

Further reading

Collins C, Roberts H, Hewer I. Anaesthesia and perioperative considerations for patients with myasthenia gravis. *AANA J*, 2020;88(6):485–491.

Gupta A, Singh-Radcliff N. *Pharmacology in Anesthesia Practice*. Oxford University Press, 2013. Anticholinesterases.

Kveraga R, Powlowski J. Anaesthesia for the Patient with Myasthenia Gravis, 2022. Available at: https://www.uptodate.com/contents/anesthesia-for-the-patient-with-myasthenia-gravis

Smith S, Scarth E. Drugs in Anaesthesia and Intensive Care, 5th edition, Oxford University Press, 2016. Neostigmine.

Thavasothy M, Hirsch N. Myasthenia gravis. *BJA CEPD Reviews*, 2002;2(3):88–90.

6. E

This scenario describes an oculogyric crisis to haloperidol. Oculogyric crises are an acute dystonia of the extraocular muscles. Features typically begin within 4 days of starting the medication or can be related to dose increases. Early signs may include restlessness and agitation followed by a fixed stare. Most usually there is fixed eye deviation upwards and laterally, but this has also been reported as a downward convergence. Other symptoms may include an arched neck, tongue protrusion, rapid blinking, lacrimation, and mutism. When caused by antipsychotic agents, features may include sweating, facial flushing, transitory hypertension, and difficulty micturating in association with hallucinations and delusions.

Other antipsychotic drugs such as prochlorperazine and olanzapine can precipitate dystonias. Other potential culprits may include metoclopramide, and selective serotonin reuptake inhibitors (SSRIs). This scenario does not describe inadequate reversal. Amisulpride is a selective dopamine antagonist (high D_2 and D_3 receptor affinity). It is typically prescribed for acute psychosis in schizophrenia; no information is presented in the scenario to support a diagnosis of schizophrenia. Additionally, administration of this drug alongside haloperidol should be avoided—both drugs prolong the QT interval and this is noted as a severe drug interaction.

Management should include discontinuation of the suspected causative agent and administration of a centrally acting antimuscarinic such as procyclidine or benzatropine intravenously. The suggested dose of IV procyclidine is 5–10 mg. Subsequent management should include consideration of further oral doses of procyclidine.

Further reading

Allman K, McIndoe A, Wilson I. *Emergencies in Anaesthesia*, 2nd edition. Oxford University Press, 2009. Neurosurgery.

Puri B, Treasden I. *Emergencies in Psychiatry*. Oxford University Press, 2008. The management of psychiatric and medical emergencies.

7. E

Sertraline is a selective serotonin (5-hydroxytryptamine) reuptake inhibitor (SSRI). They are probably the most widely used group of antidepressants in use. Other SSRIs include fluoxetine, paroxetine, and citalopram.

They have a generally favourable side effect profile in comparison to other groups of antidepressants. Side effects may include a rise or fall in heart rate, hypotension, hyponatraemia, nausea, abdominal pain, and hypersensitivity. They are extensively metabolized by the hepatic cytochrome P450 system and renally excreted. Many antidepressants are associated with hyponatraemia, however, the highest risk is with SSRIs. Consideration should be given to selecting an alternative such as a tricyclic antidepressant (TCA) or MAOI if severe. Altered taste has been reported with sertraline, amitriptyline, and bupropion.

Studies suggest SSRIs are associated with an increased risk of bleeding, however the overall chance of experiencing a significant event is rare. The proposed mechanism is the inhibition of the uptake of serotonin into platelets, leading to platelet dysfunction and reduced effectiveness of normal clotting processes. They are potent inhibitors of cytochrome p450, so vigilance with co-administration of other drugs metabolized by these enzyme systems is required.

Abrupt cessation of many antidepressant drugs can lead to a withdrawal or discontinuation syndrome. SSRIs, tricyclic antidepressants (TCAs), monoamine oxidase inhibitors (MAOIs), selective noradrenaline reuptake inhibitors (e.g. duloxetine), and various atypical agents such as mirtazapine, venlafaxine, and trazodone have all been associated with this potential syndrome. Symptoms typically include insomnia, hyperarousal, nausea, balance disruption, and flu-like symptoms. Appropriate gradual tapering of doses should be undertaken and patient education is key.

Tricyclic antidepressants (TCAs; for example, amitriptyline) selectively inhibit the presynaptic reuptake of noradrenaline (and variably among different agents, serotonin). Monoamine oxidase inhibitors (MAOIs; for example, isocarboxazid) bind to mitochondrial monoamine oxidase increasing the concentration of monoamines within the CNS. Both TCAs and MAOIs have potentially significant side effects and toxicity profiles when compared with SSRIs.

Other antidepressant drugs include trazodone (which is a mixed serotonin receptor agonist/antagonist) and bupropion (which is a weak noradrenaline and dopamine uptake inhibitor and can be prescribed for its antidepressant effects or to support smoking cessation).

Further reading

Gelder M, Andreasen N, Lopez-Ibor J, Geddes J. *New Oxford Textbook of Psychiatry*, 2nd edition. Oxford University Press, 2012. Antidepressants.

Ereshefsky L, Riesenman C, Lam YWF. Antidepressant drug interactions and the cytochrome P450 system. *Clin Pharmacokinet*, 1995;29:10–19.

Smith S, Scarth E. *Drugs in Anaesthesia and Intensive Care*, 5th edition. Oxford University Press, 2016. Amitriptylin, Phenelzine, SSRIs.

Drugs affecting the cardiovascular system

QUESTIONS

Multiple-Choice Questions

1. Which of the following drugs antagonize alpha adrenoceptors?

A Clonidine

B Labetalol

C Phentolamine

D Phenylephrine

E Tamsulosin

2. A 45-year-old female patient presents to the preoperative assessment clinic the day before she is scheduled to have a vaginal hysterectomy. Her lowest blood pressure (BP) measured is 165/90. Which actions should be taken?

A Start an angiotensin-converting enzyme (ACE) inhibitor (ACEi)

B Continue with surgery

C Inform GP

D Start metoprolol

E Refer the patient to the medical on-call team

3. Drugs that can cause a reduction in systemic vascular resistance

A Dobutamine

B Dopamine

C Levosimendan

D Milrinone

E Noradrenaline

4. Clonidine

A Acts on post-synaptic alpha-2 receptors

B Can cause a transient increase in blood pressure

C Prolongs duration of local anaesthesia when co-administered for neural blockade

D Elimination half-life is reduced in renal impairment

E Oral bioavailability is 100%

5. A 33-year-old banker has been brought into the emergency department by his friends who were celebrating with him after the conclusion of an important deal. He is acutely agitated and confused with a blood pressure of 200/110. They say no alcohol was consumed but one witnessed the patient snorting 'something'. Which drugs would be beneficial in managing this case?

A Labetalol 50 mg IV

B 50 ml of mannitol 20% IV

C Nimodipine sublingually

D Ramipril 5 mg orally

E Sodium nitroprusside infusion

6. Adrenaline

A Has enantiomers

B Will increase insulin requirements in diabetic patients

C 5 ml 1:1000 nebulized is appropriate for a one-year-old baby with croup

D Dose should be limited to 5 mcg/kg/30 mins in the presence of isoflurane

E 0.3 ml 1:1000 IM is appropriate management for an eight-year-old child in anaphylaxis

7. In pregnancy

A ACEi are safe to continue in the management of chronic hypertension

B Patients with type 1 diabetes should be taking 75 mg aspirin daily from 12 weeks

C Patients with gestational hypertension and blood pressure 145/95 mmHg should be treated with oral labetalol

D Pre-eclamptic patients with blood pressure 145/95 mmHg should be admitted to hospital

E Pre-eclamptic patients with blood pressure 145/95 mmHg should be treated with oral labetalol

Single Best Answers

1.
A 73-year-old male patient arrives at the pre-op assessment clinic. He is scheduled for a hiatus hernia repair tomorrow. Initial observations show a respiratory rate of 18 breaths per minute, oxygen saturation of 97% on room air, blood pressure of 110/70 mmHg, and a heart rate of 160 beats per minute. The nurse brings you the electrocardiograph (ECG) which shows a broad complex tachycardia. What is the most appropriate management?

A Adenosine 6 mg IV

B Amiodarone 300 mg IV

C Lidocaine 100 mg IV

D Sotolol 100 mg IV

E Synchronized DC cardioversion

2.
A 68-year-old male patient monitored in cardiac intensive care, 4 hours after coronary artery bypass surgery, enters witnessed ventricular fibrillation (VF). The most appropriate initial management is?

A Adrenaline 1 mg IM

B Amiodarone 300 mg IV

C Deliver up to three stacked direct current (DC) shocks

D Initiate open chest protocol

E Start cardiopulmonary resuscitation (CPR) with DC shock as soon as possible

3. A 62-year-old male patient scheduled for a left total knee replacement next week attends pre-op assessment clinic. His best BP of three is recorded as 170/115. He is known to be hypertensive and his regular medications include amlodipine 10 mg OD and candesartan 16 mg OD. What would be the most appropriate next step in his management?

A He can continue to surgery with GP follow-up post-op

B Refer back to the GP, who will add in bendroflumethiazide

C Refer back to the GP, who will add in indapamide

D Refer back to the GP, who will switch candesartan to ramipril

E Start atenolol now and continue to surgery as planned

4. A 22-year-old male patient is being managed on the neuro intensive care unit (ICU) with a severe traumatic brain injury. He is becoming progressively more tachycardic with a heart rate of 120 bpm. His BP is 95/60 mmHg despite aggressive fluid filling and his urine output has been greater than 500 ml/hr for the last two hours. Which of the following infusions would you start?

A Adrenaline

B Dobutamine

C Metaraminol

D Noradrenaline

E Vasopressin

5. An 18-month-old child has been admitted to the ICU with sepsis. She has had 60 ml/kg in total of IV isotonic saline and a dopamine infusion has been started, running at 10 mcg/kg/min. She is peripherally cold and mottled, with a central capillary refill time (CRT) of four seconds. Her blood pressure is 80/50. What is your next step for managing her septic shock?

A Add in an adrenaline infusion

B Add in a milrinone infusion

C Add in a noradrenaline infusion

D Give a 20 ml/kg bolus IV 5% albumin

E Start a vasopressin infusion

6. A 38-year-old man, who is paraplegic with a T4 spinal cord injury he acquired in his 20s, is in the post-anaesthesia care unit (PACU) recovering from a laparoscopic cholecystectomy. You have been called to see him as his blood pressure has suddenly risen to 220/115 mmHg. He is complaining of a headache and appears flushed and sweaty. After ensuring his urinary catheter is patent and his rectum is empty, what would you do?

A Administer 1–2 tablets of glyceryl trinitrate (GTN) sublingually

B Give hydralazine 20 mg IV

C Give labetalol 20 mg IV

D Start a magnesium sulfate infusion

E Start an IV GTN infusion

7. A 53-year-old female patient with asymptomatic hypertrophic cardiomyopathy (HCM) has a general anaesthetic for a total abdominal hysterectomy. Shortly after induction, her blood pressure falls to 90/55. What is the best way to manage this situation?

A 500 ml IV fluid bolus and phenylephrine infusion

B Incremental 10 mcg boluses of adrenaline

C Insert a central line and start a noradrenaline infusion

D Obtain a transoesophageal echocardiogram (TOE)

E Reduce the depth of anaesthetic

ANSWERS

Multiple-Choice Questions

1. FTTFT

Clonidine is an alpha-2 adrenoceptor agonist. Phenylephrine is a direct alpha-1 agonist. Labetalol is a selective alpha-1, beta-1, and beta-2 adrenoceptor antagonist. Phentolamine is a competitive alpha antagonist. Tamsulosin is a selective alpha-1 antagonist used in benign prostatic hypertrophy.

Further reading

Scarth E, Smith S. *Drugs in Anaesthesia and Intensive Care*, 5th edition. Oxford University Press, 2016. Clonidine, Labetalol, Phentolamine, Phenylephrine.

2. FTTFF

The GP referral to the surgeon should include documented evidence of blood pressure recordings below 160/100 mmHg in the last year. If the blood pressure is being assessed in a secondary care environment (i.e. pre-op assessment clinic), then blood pressure less than 180/110 mmHg is acceptable to proceed. The GP should, however, still be informed of readings in excess of 140/90 mmHg so that the diagnosis of hypertension can be confirmed, investigated, and treated as necessary. Starting antihypertensives the day before surgery is not appropriate and any such interventions should also be managed by the patient's GP.

Further reading

Hartle A, et al. AAGBI Guideline: The measurement of adult blood pressure and management of hypertension before elective surgery. *Anaesthesia*, 2016;17:326–337.

Smith S, Scarth E. *Drugs in Anaesthesia and Intensive Care*, 5th edition. Oxford University Press, 2016. ACE inhibitors.

3. TTTTF

At low doses (5 mcg/kg/min) the beta-adrenergic effects of dopamine are predominant. The beta-2 effect may lead to a reduction in systemic vascular resistance. Dobutamine also has a direct beta-2 agonist effect. Levosimendan is a calcium sensitizer, but also stimulates ATP-dependent K channels, leading to vasodilatation. Milrinone is a selective phosphodiesterase III inhibitor in cardiac and vascular muscle. It causes cAMP-dependent protein phosphorylation and subsequent vascular muscle relaxation. The primary action of noradrenaline is increasing systemic vascular resistance by acting at alpha-adrenergic receptors.

Further reading

Scarth E, Smith S. *Drugs in Anaesthesia and Intensive Care*, 5th edition. Oxford University Press, 2016. Dobutamine, Dopamine, Levosimendan, Milrinone, Noradrenaline.

4. FTTFT

Clonidine stimulates pre-synaptic alpha-2 adrenoceptors, reducing noradrenaline release and thereby decreasing sympathetic tone. Dexmedetomidine acts on post-synaptic alpha-2 receptors. When administered IV, clonidine stimulates vascular alpha-1 receptors and causes a transient increase in blood pressure. The drug is absorbed rapidly when administered orally with a bioavailability of 100%. 65% of clonidine is excreted unchanged in the urine. The dose should be reduced if the eGFR is less than 10ml/min. Clonidine cannot be removed by haemodialysis.

Further reading

Scarth E, Smith S. *Drugs in Anaesthesia and Intensive Care*, 5th edition. Oxford University Press, 2016. Clonidine, Appendix A1.3.

5. TFFFT

This patient has hypertensive encephalopathy caused by a sudden, sustained rise in blood pressure exceeding the upper limit of cerebral autoregulation. Likely secondary to cocaine use. The primary aim of therapy is prompt, titratable, lowering of arterial blood pressure. For this, short-acting IV agents and infusions are the most useful.

Sodium nitroprusside (SNP) is a very fast-acting and titratable vasodilator which acts to stabilize the smooth muscle cell membrane by interacting with sulfhydryl groups and preventing calcium influx necessary for contraction. Unfortunately, SNP has the potential to cause cyanide toxicity at higher rates of infusion. At higher plasma concentrations, the drug is metabolized by rapid non-enzymatic hydrolysis in red blood cells. By this mechanism, each SNP molecule produces five cyanide ions. The management of cyanide ion toxicity includes administering either sodium thiosulphate or dicobalt edetate.

Labetalol is a non-selective beta-antagonist with 7:1 beta:alpha activity. Its antihypertensive effect is primarily through a reduction in peripheral vascular resistance while cardiac output and heart rate are maintained. It is the combined adrenergic antagonism that makes this drug especially useful in times of catecholamine excess, such as this case. The onset of action is within 2–15 minutes when administered IV and may last up to 6 hours. The BNF (British National Formulary) recommends a dose of 50 mg over 1 minute to be repeated at 5 min intervals up to a maximum dose of 200 mg.

Mannitol is an osmotic diuretic widely used in the management of raised intracerebral pressure and cerebral oedema. A dose of 0.25–2 g/kg is recommended by the BNF. The dose stated here (10 g) is therefore a significant underdosing. Sublingual nimodipine will have a rapid onset of action, but is uncontrollable and can have serious adverse effects including cerebral ischaemia and myocardial infarction. Ramipril has a time to peak effect of 3–6 hours with its antihypertensive effect lasting for 24 hours. It is therefore neither fast-acting, nor titratable, and therefore also inappropriate in this circumstance.

Further reading

Lamy C, Mas JL. Hypertensive encephalopathy. In Grotta JC, et al. (eds) *Stroke*, 6th edition. Elsevier, 2016. Pages 640–647.

Scarth E, Smith S. *Drugs in Anaesthesia and Intensive Care*, 5th edition. Oxford University Press, 2016. ACE inhibitors, Mannitol, Nimodipine, Sodium Nitroprusside.

6. TTTFT

Adrenaline is a racemic 1:1 mixture of dextro and levo rotatory enantiomers. The D-type has approximately 1/12th to 1/18th of the potency of the levo form. L-adrenaline is available as an enantiopure preparation. Adrenaline increases plasma blood glucose, reduces endogenous insulin secretion, and increases the rate of glycogenolysis. Diabetic patients may require dose increases of their insulin.

Doses should be limited to 3 mcg/kg/30 mins in the presence of isoflurane (or 1 mcg/kg/30 mins for halothane) due to the risk of precipitating severe ventricular dysrhythmias. Paediatric IM doses of 1:1000 adrenaline doses for anaphylaxis are: child age <6 years = 0.15 ml (150 mcg), child age 6–12 years = 0.3 ml (300 mcg) and children >12 years = as per adult algorithm 0.5 ml (500 mcg).

Further reading

Resuscitation Council UK. Available at: https://www.resus.org.uk/

Scarth E, Smith S. *Drugs in Anaesthesia and Intensive Care*, 5th edition. Oxford University Press, 2016. Adrenaline, Insulin, Isoflurane.

7. FTFTF

Pregnant patients with type 1 diabetes are at high risk of pre-eclampsia, and therefore should take daily aspirin from 12 weeks. Other high-risk factors for pre-eclampsia include:

- Hypertensive disease during a previous pregnancy
- Chronic kidney disease
- Autoimmune disease
- Type 2 diabetes
- Chronic hypertension

For a patient with gestational hypertension, a blood pressure of 145/95 mmHg is regarded as mild, and therefore does not need admission or treatment. For a patient with pre-eclampsia, however, a blood pressure of 145/95 mmHg requires admission to hospital, but not treatment. ACE inhibitors and angiotensin receptor blockers (ARBs) are associated with an increased risk of congenital abnormalities if taken during pregnancy.

Further reading

NICE. Hypertension in Pregnancy: Diagnosis and Management [CG107], 2010. Available at: https://www.nice.org.uk/guidance/cg107

Smith S, Scarth E. *Drugs in Anaesthesia and Intensive Care*, 5th edition. Oxford University Press, 2016. ACE inhibitors, Aspirin, Magnesium.

Single Best Answers

1. B

As per the Resuscitation Council UK 2015 guidelines for tachycardia. The patient shows no adverse signs which would lead to a synchronized shock. Adenosine or sotalol could be considered if it were a narrow complex tachycardia. This could, of course, be a regular narrow complex tachycardia with a bundle branch block, but without knowing that the patient has pre-existing bundle branch block from previous ECGs, it should be assumed to be a new broad complex tachycardia.

Further reading

Resuscitation Council UK. Adult Tachycardia Algorithm, 2015. Available at: https://www.resus.org.uk/sites/default/files/2021-04/Tachycardia%20Algorithm%202021.pdf

Smith S, Scarth E. *Drugs in Anaesthesia and Intensive Care*, 5th edition. Oxford University Press, 2016. Adenosine, Amiodarone, Lidocaine.

2. C

The cardiac advanced life support algorithm states that if the ECG shows VF or pulseless ventricular tachycardia (VT) then external cardiac massage can be delayed up to 1 minute to administer up to three consecutive DC shocks. After cardiac surgery chest compressions are associated with potentially fatal complications and may not be necessary. The likelihood of success declines significantly with sequential shocks (78% —> 35% —> 14%) and therefore resternotomy would be preferable to performing a fourth shock. Adrenaline administration is not a part of the cardiac ALS protocol. Amiodarone may be helpful at a later time, but is not the best initial management.

Further reading

Smith S, Scarth E. *Drugs in Anaesthesia and Intensive Care*, 5th edition. Oxford University Press, 2016. Adrenaline, Amiodarone.

Society of Thoracic Surgeons Task Force on Resuscitation After Cardiac Surgery. The Society of Thoracic Surgeons expert consensus for the resuscitation of patients who arrest after cardiac surgery. *Ann Thoracic Surg*, 2017;103:1005–1020.

3. C

After three readings, the lowest systolic BP should be below 180 mmHg AND the lowest diastolic BP below 110 mmHg in order for elective surgery to proceed as planned with GP follow-up post-op. This patient would fit into the category of step 3 treatment, which involves the addition of a thiazide-like diuretic, such as indapamide. The GP should be the one to start new antihypertensive medications, not the pre-op assessment clinic. Non-cancer elective surgery should be delayed for a minimum of six weeks to allow new antihypertensive medication to be established and a sustained improvement in BP achieved.

Further reading

Hartle A, et al. AAGBI Guideline: the measurement of adult blood pressure and management of hypertension before elective surgery. *Anaesthesia*, 2016;17:326–337.

Smith S, Scarth E. *Drugs in Anaesthesia and Intensive Care*, 5th edition. Oxford University Press, 2016. ACE inhibitors, Amlodipine, A2RA, Bendroflumethiazide.

4. E

Cardiovascular instability is common in the patient with a severe traumatic brain injury progressing to brainstem death. Contributing factors include loss of vasomotor tone secondary to catecholamine depletion, diabetes insipidus (DI) secondary to acute posterior pituitary failure and myocardial depression secondary to catecholamine and cytokine toxicity. Early restoration of vascular tone can reduce the risks of excessive fluid administration. Vasopressin is considered the first-line agent in this situation as it:

- Restores vasomotor tone
- Treats DI
- Minimizes catecholamine requirements
- Is less likely than noradrenaline to cause metabolic acidosis or pulmonary hypertension.

Vasopressin (8-arginine-vasopressin) is a synthetic nonapeptide, identical to human endogenous vasopressin (antidiuretic hormone). It has actions on multiple receptors via G-protein linked receptors (V1; vascular smooth muscle constriction. V2; renal control of plasma volume and osmolality, V3; pituitary release of ACTH) and exhibits the same affinity as oxytocin for binding to oxytocin type receptors. Dosing is independent of hepatic and renal function.

Further reading

Gordon J, et al. Physiological changes after brain stem death and management of the heart beating donor. *Cont Educ Anaesth Crit Care Pain*, 2012;12(5):225–229.

Sharman A, Low J. Vasopressin and its role in critical care. *Cont Educ Anaesth Crit Care Pain*, 2008;8(4):134–137.

Smith S, Scarth E. *Drugs in Anaesthesia and Intensive Care*, 5th edition. Oxford University Press, 2016. Adrenaline, Dobutamine, Metaraminol, Noradrenaline, Vasopressin.

5. A

This patient has cold shock. She is fluid and dopamine resistant. The next step in the paediatric sepsis algorithm is to start an adrenaline infusion. Noradrenaline or vasopressin would be the choice for warm shock. Milrinone would be the correct choice if she had cold shock with a normal blood pressure. In 'cold shock' there is typically low cardiac output, high systemic vascular resistance, and cool shut-down peripheries. 'Warm shock', by contrast, describes high cardiac output, low systemic vascular resistance, and peripheral vasodilation with bounding pulses. Inadequate tissue perfusion is common in both forms.

Further reading

Brierley J, et al. Clinical practice parameters for haemodynamic support of paediatric and neonatal septic shock: 2007 update from the American College of Critical Care Medicine. *Crit Care Med*, 2009;37:666–688.

Smith S, Scarth E. *Drugs in Anaesthesia and Intensive Care*, 5th edition. Oxford University Press, 2016. Adrenaline, Dopamine, Human albumin solution, Milrinone, Noradrenaline, Vasopressin.

6. A

This man is experiencing autonomic dysreflexia. It is a medical emergency resulting in severe hypertension following a disordered autonomic response to stimuli below the level of the spinal cord injury. Incidence is 50–70% in patients with a spinal cord lesion above T6. The most common triggers are bladder distension and constipation, which is why these are checked first. Initial pharmacological management should be sublingual GTN or nifedipine. Both are fast-acting, easy to administer, and readily available in a hospital environment. It is often associated with a bradycardia reflex, and therefore labetalol would not be the best choice. Hydralazine, magnesium, and IV GTN would all be considered as subsequent management options.

Further reading

Petsas A, Drake J. Perioperative management for patients with a chronic spinal cord injury. *BJA Education*, 2015;15(3):123–130.

Royal College of Physicians British Society of Rehabilitation Medicine, Multidisciplinary Association of Spinal Cord Injury Professionals, British

Association of Spinal Cord Injury Professionals, British Association of Spinal Injury Specialists, and Spinal Injuries Association. A Series of Evidence-Based Guidelines for Clinical Management: Guideline Number 9: Chronic Spinal Cord Injury: Management of Patients in Acute Hospital Settings. Royal College of Physicians, 2008. Available at: https://www.bsrm.org.uk/downloads/sciwebversion.pdf

Smith S, Scarth E. *Drugs in Anaesthesia and Intensive Care*, 5th edition. Oxford University Press, 2016. Glyceryl trinitrate, Hydralazine, Magnesium.

7. A

In the management of patients with HCM, the aim is to:

- Maintain sinus rhythm
- Keep sympathetic activity to a minimum to reduce chronotropy and inotropy
- Maintain left ventricular filling
- Maintain systemic vascular resistance (SVR).

In this case, it is likely that at induction, the patient who is relatively underfilled due to being fasted pre-op, has a drop in her SVR and goes on to develop left ventricular outflow tract (LVOT) obstruction. It would be ideal to obtain a TOE to formalize this diagnosis, however she must be managed while this is organized and treatment should be commenced immediately. Answers A and C will both lead to increased sympathetic activity and therefore be detrimental to her condition.

Further reading

Davies MR, Cousins J. Cardiomyopathy and anaesthesia. *Cont Educ Crit Care Pain*, 2009;9(6):189–193.

Smith S, Scarth E. *Drugs in Anaesthesia and Intensive Care*, 5th edition. Oxford University Press, 2016. Adrenaline, Noradrenaline, Phenylephrine.

Drugs affecting the respiratory system

QUESTIONS

Multiple-Choice Questions

1. Recognized treatments for pulmonary arterial hypertension include:

A Warfarin

B Nebulized iloprost

C Digoxin

D Oxygen

E Pulmonary endarterectomy

2. In a patient suffering from acute severe asthma, it is appropriate to administer:

A Oxygen to maintain SpO_2 88–92%

B IV β_2 agonist

C Nebulized β_2 agonist

D Nebulized magnesium sulfate

E IV antibiotics

3. In the management of asthma during pregnancy, the following should be used as they would be in non-pregnant patients:

A Oral theophylline

B Short-acting β_2 agonist

C Oral steroids

D Inhaled corticosteroids

E Long-acting β_2 agonist

4. The following techniques can be used in the management of theophylline poisoning:

A Encourage vomiting

B Ondansetron

C Haemodialysis

D Activated charcoal

E Potassium chloride

5. Regarding long-term oxygen therapy (LTOT), which of the following statements are correct?

A Supplemental oxygen needs to be breathed for at least 15 hours day^{-1} to improve mortality

B The mortality benefit of LTOT comes from reducing pulmonary arterial pressure

C LTOT is only effective if, with it, oxygen saturations are maintained >92%

D LTOT is indicated in stable chronic obstructive pulmonary disease (COPD) patients with PaO$_2$ <8 and peripheral oedema

E LTOT can be used to treat isolated nocturnal hypoxaemia caused by COPD

6. The following effects are associated with the use of high oxygen concentrations:

A Pulmonary congestion

B Increased cerebral blood flow

C Increased vital capacity

D Reduced cardiac output

E Altered lymphocyte production

7. Salbutamol

A Is an agonist at the beta-1 adrenoceptor

B Crosses the placenta and can cause foetal tachycardia

C Causes a rise in plasma potassium concentration

D Potentiates the action of non-depolarizing muscle relaxants

E Can cause lactic acidosis

Single Best Answers

1. A 28-year-old primiparous woman is having a category 2 caesarean section for failure to progress at 39/40. She does not report any significant medical history and has had an uncomplicated pregnancy to date. She has a spinal anaesthetic, which is working well. Following the delivery of a healthy baby, she suffers a severe post-postpartum haemorrhage (PPH) due to uterine atony. She begins to complain of shortness of breath and her oxygen saturation begins to drop. What is the most likely cause?

A Amniotic fluid embolus

B Carboprost

C Ergometrine

D High spinal

E Oxytocin

2. A 32-year-old man has undergone an open appendicectomy. His only past medical history is a diagnosis of testicular cancer for which he had previously received bleomycin and had surgery with curative intent. He takes no regular medications now and has no known allergies. On the day 1 postoperative ward round he is noted to be dyspnoeic with pleuritic chest pain and a dry cough. His oxygen saturations are 94% on 4 litres min^{-1} oxygen delivered by nasal cannulae. What is the most important action to take?

A Give therapeutic low molecular weight heparin

B Increase administered oxygen to target saturations of 98%

C Remove supplementary oxygen

D Request a chest X-ray

E Take an arterial blood sample

3. A 26-year-old female presents four months after a lung transplant for cystic fibrosis with dyspnoea, hypoxia, and lethargy. She denies any cough. Her respiratory rate is 32 min^{-1}, oxygen saturation 92% on 10 L/min^{-1} O$_2$, heart rate 100 min^{-1}, blood pressure 96/58 mmHg, and temperature is 37.1°C. Her chest X-ray shows bilateral diffuse infiltrates. Given the likely diagnosis, what is the most important therapy?

A Diagnostic bronchoscopy

B Increase FiO$_2$

C IV amoxicillin and clarithromycin

D Nebulized amphotericin

E Pulsed methylprednisolone

4. A 70 kg, 54-year-old man has been intubated and ventilated in an intensive care unit (ICU) for three days. He is influenza positive. His chest radiograph shows diffuse bilateral pulmonary infiltrates. He has an increasing oxygen requirement and currently his FiO_2 is 0.8 with pH 7.22, PaO_2 8 kPa, and $PaCO_2$ 6.4 kPa. He is on volume-controlled ventilation with PEEP 8 cmH$_2$O, respiratory rate 20 min^{-1}, and tidal volume 500 ml. What should be the next step in optimizing his respiratory function prior to referral for extracorporeal membrane oxygenation (ECMO)?

A Exogenous surfactant replacement

B Inhaled nitric oxide

C Inhaled prostacyclin

D IV methylprednisolone

E Reduce tidal volume to 420 ml

5. A 32/40 pregnant woman is seen in the emergency department. She has been sent in by her midwife who is concerned about her breathing following a routine appointment. She appears to be breathless at rest, using her accessory muscles and is somewhat anxious. She can speak short sentences and says that aside from the breathlessness she feels well in herself. Her observations are: respiratory rate 32 min^{-1}; saturations on room air 92%; blood pressure 124/60 mmHg; heart rate 110 min^{-1}; and temperature 37.3°C. Given the most likely diagnosis, what is the most appropriate action?

A Give IV co-amoxiclav

B Give treatment dose low molecular weight heparin

C Request compression duplex ultrasound

D Request CT pulmonary angiogram (CTPA)

E Start IV unfractionated heparin infusion

6. You have been asked to help in the management of a 14-month-old boy who has presented to the emergency department with a barking cough. His mother describes a two-day history of coryzal symptoms with his symptoms getting much worse tonight. On examination, he is agitated with moderate inspiratory stridor (which Mum says is there at rest, too), intercostal recession, reduced air entry throughout and saturations of 88% on room air. After delivering oxygen, what action should be taken?

A Gently use a tongue depressor to see inside the mouth for any causes of upper airway obstruction

B Give 2 mg nebulized budesonide

C Give 5 ml 1:1000 nebulized adrenaline

D Give oral dexamethasone 0.15 mg/kg

E Insert an IV cannula and give IV hydrocortisone

7. You anaesthetize a 68-year-old man for a hip replacement. He is normally well except for severe gastro-oesophageal reflux disease and osteoarthritis. He has no known allergies and has never had a problem with anaesthetics. He refused a regional anaesthetic and because of his reflux disease, you performed a rapid sequence induction with suxamethonium. The standard antibiotic prophylaxis for this operation is teicoplanin and gentamicin, so you give those before surgery. Shortly after the surgeons make their incision, the patient's oxygen saturations fall and he becomes very difficult to ventilate with high airway pressures. He has significant bronchospasm on auscultation and you determine that he is having an anaphylactic reaction. What is the most likely causative agent?

A Atracurium

B Chlorhexidine

C Gentamicin

D Suxamethonium

E Teicoplanin

ANSWERS

Multiple-Choice Questions

1. TTTTF

Pulmonary hypertension is defined as a mean pulmonary arterial pressure (MPAP) ≥25 mmHg at rest or 30 mmHg on exercise.

Pulmonary endarterectomy is only a valid treatment option specifically for chronic thromboembolic pulmonary hypertension (CTEPH). It is not a treatment for other forms of pulmonary arterial hypertension (PAH). Diuretics are useful in the presence of heart failure or raised right atrial pressure. Iloprost is a prostacyclin analogue commonly used to treat pulmonary hypertension in the UK.

Further reading

Elliot CA, et al. Pulmonary hypertension. *Cont Educ Anaesth Crit Care Pain*, 2006;6 (1):17–22.

Smith S, Scarth E. *Drugs in Anaesthesia and Intensive Care*, 5th edition. Oxford University Press, 2016. Epoprostenol, Oxygen.

2. FFTFF

Acute severe asthma is categorized by the presence of any one of:

PEF 33–50% best or predicted
Respiratory rate ≥ 25 min^{-1}
Heart rate ≥ 110 min^{-1}

Inability to complete sentences in one breath

The oxygen saturation target for hypoxaemic patients suffering from acute severe asthma is 94–98%. IV β_2 agonists should be reserved for patients in whom inhaled therapy cannot be used reliably. High-dose inhaled β_2 agonists delivered by oxygen-driven nebulizers should be used as the first-line agents. A single dose of IV magnesium sulfate can be used in patients who do not have a good response to inhaled bronchodilator therapy. Nebulized magnesium is not recommended. Routine use of IV antibiotics is also not recommended in acute asthma.

Further reading

British Thoracic Society. British Guideline on the Management of Asthma. QRG 153, 2016. Available at: https://www.brit-thoracic.org.uk/document-library/guidelines/asthma/btssign-asthma-guideline-quick-reference-guide-2016

Smith S, Scarth E. *Drugs in Anaesthesia and Intensive Care*, 5th edition. Oxford University Press, 2016. Magnesium, Salbutamol.

3. **TTTTT**

Physiological changes in pregnancy can worsen or improve asthma. It is important for women to maintain good control of their asthma during pregnancy to avoid problems for themselves and their baby. All drug therapies for asthma should be used in pregnant patients as they would be for non-pregnant patients.

Further reading

British Thoracic Society. British Guideline on the Management of Asthma. QRG 153, 2016. Available at: https://www.brit-thoracic. org.uk/document-library/guidelines/asthma/btssign-asthma-guidel ine-quick-reference-guide-2016

Smith S, Scarth E. *Drugs in Anaesthesia and Intensive Care*, 5th edition. Oxford University Press, 2016. Aminophylline, Prednisolone, Salbutamol.

4. **FTFTT**

Theophylline and related drugs are often prescribed in modified-release formats. Therefore the symptoms of toxicity are often delayed.

Symptoms include:

Vomiting
Agitation
Restlessness
Dilated pupils
Tachycardia
Convulsions

Hypokalaemia

Vomiting should not be encouraged, rather it should be managed with antiemetics such as ondansetron. Hypokalaemia may occur rapidly, so must be closely monitored and managed with potassium chloride infusion. Activated charcoal may be used to eliminate theophylline even if more than one hour has passed since ingestion.

Further reading

Smith S, Scarth E. *Drugs in Anaesthesia and Intensive Care*, 5th edition. Oxford University Press, 2016. Aminophylline.

5. **TTFTF**

For LTOT to be effective in prolonging life, it must be used for >15 hours day^{-1} with oxygen saturations maintained >90%. It is indicated in stable patients with PaO_2 >7.3 kPa or between 7.3 kPa and 8.0 kPa if they have one or more of:

- Polycythaemia
- Peripheral oedema
- Pulmonary hypertension

NICE guidance states that LTOT should not be offered to patients with isolated nocturnal hypoxaemia caused by COPD.

Further reading

Lumb A, Biercamp C. Chronic obstructive pulmonary disease and anaesthesia. *Cont Educ Anaesth Crit Care Pain*, 2014;14(1):1–5.

NICE. Chronic Obstructive Pulmonary Disease in Over 16s: Diagnosis and Management [NG115], 2018. Available at: https://www.nice.org.uk/guidance/ng115

Smith S, Scarth E. *Drugs in Anaesthesia and Intensive Care*, 5th edition. Oxford University Press, 2016. Oxygen.

6. TFFTF

Oxygen is the most widely used drug in anaesthesia and critical care. However, there is increasing doubt around the presumed benefits of hyperoxia and even maintaining normoxaemia during critical illness.

Within 2–3 minutes of breathing 100% O_2, nitrogen is eliminated from the lungs, which leads to atelectasis and a reduction in vital capacity, secondary to the loss of the 'splinting' effect. 100% oxygen causes cerebrovascular vasoconstriction which results in a decrease in cerebral blood flow. High oxygen concentrations cause reduced cardiac output from 8 to 20% due to myocardial depression. Administration of 100% oxygen may also interfere with red blood cell formation. Hyperoxia causes an inflammatory response and cellular damage through the production of reactive oxygen intermediates. This inflammatory response can cause pulmonary congestion and a picture similar to acute respiratory distress syndrome (ARDS).

Further reading

Martin DS, Grocott MPW III. Oxygen therapy in anaesthesia: the yin and yang of O_2. *Br J Anaesth*, 2013;111(6):867–871.

Smith S, Scarth E. *Drugs in Anaesthesia and Intensive Care*, 5th edition. Oxford University Press, 2016. Oxygen.

7. TTFTT

Salbutamol is a beta-adrenergic agonist with greater activity at beta-2 receptors than beta-1. In high doses, the beta-1 actions lead to positive inotropic and chronotropic effects. The drug reduces the tone of the gravid uterus and 10% of an administered dose will cross the placenta and can lead to foetal side effects. Salbutamol causes a drop in the plasma potassium concentration by shifting the ion intracellularly. Anxiety, insomnia, tremor, sweating, palpitations, ketosis, lactic acidosis, hypokalaemia, postural hypotension, and nausea and vomiting may occur following use of the drug.

Further reading

Smith S, Scarth E. *Drugs in Anaesthesia and Intensive Care*, 5th edition. Oxford University Press, 2016. Salbutamol.

Single Best Answers

1. B

Given the history of PPH, it is more likely that her shortness of breath has been caused by a drug given as part of the PPH management protocol than an amniotic fluid embolus. At this stage in her procedure, we would expect the level of her spinal anaesthetic to be lowering, therefore answer D is also unlikely. Cough, respiratory disorders, and chest discomfort are all listed in the BNF (British National Formulary) as side effects of carboprost. It is contraindicated in asthmatic patients.

Further reading

Smith S, Scarth E. *Drugs in Anaesthesia and Intensive Care*, 5th edition. Oxford University Press, 2016. Oxytocin.

2. C

Bleomycin is a cytotoxic antibiotic used as chemotherapy for germ cell tumours and Hodgkin's disease. Pulmonary toxicity can occur in 6–10% of patients and can be fatal. Importantly, for the anaesthetist, even short periods of high inspired oxygen concentrations are implicated in rapidly progressing pulmonary toxicity. This is the case even in patients who are no longer taking bleomycin but have been exposed in the past. Supplemental oxygen should not be given except in an emergency to keep saturations at 88–92%.

Further reading

Allan N, et al. Anaesthetic implications of chemotherapy. *Cont Educ Anaesth Crit Care Pain*, 2012;12(2):52–56.

Smith S, Scarth E. *Drugs in Anaesthesia and Intensive Care*, 5th edition. Oxford University Press, 2016. Oxygen.

3. E

This patient has acute graft rejection. Over a third of all lung transplant recipients will develop acute rejection in the first year after transplant. The most obvious differential is respiratory sepsis. The patient does not have a spontaneous cough because the lung is denervated and the cough reflex lost. A diagnostic bronchoscopy would be useful but not therapeutic. Antibiotics should be given, but IV amoxicillin and clarithromycin would not be the best choice for an immunosuppressed patient. Nebulized amphotericin is used post-op in lung transplant as fungal prophylaxis but is not the most important therapy here. The FiO$_2$ delivered should be titrated to arterial blood gas results. Increasing immunosuppression with pulsed methylprednisolone is the treatment of choice for acute rejection.

Further reading

Allman K, Wilson I, O'Donnell A. *Oxford Handbook of Anaesthesia*, 4th edition. Oxford University Press, 2016.

Fitzgerald M, Ryan D. Cystic fibrosis and anaesthesia. *Cont Educ Anaesth Crit Care Pain*, 2011;11(6):204–209.

Nickson C. Lung Transplant. *Life in the Fast Lane (liftl.com)*, 2019. Available at: https://litfl.com/lung-transplant/

Smith S, Scarth E. *Drugs in Anaesthesia and Intensive Care*, 5th edition. Oxford University Press, 2016. Amphotericin.

4. E

All of these strategies have been implemented at various times in the management of ARDS. However, the only strategy that has a strong evidence base for improving outcomes is protective ventilation with <6 ml/kg tidal volumes and plateau pressures <30 cmH$_2$O. An inability to achieve lung-protective tidal volumes and pressures is part of the ECMO referral criteria.

Further reading

Mackay A, Al-Haddad M. Acute lung injury and acute respiratory distress syndrome. *Cont Educ in Anaesth Crit Care Pain*, 2009;9(5):152–156.

Royal Brompton. ECMO Referral and Transfer Pathway, 2022. Available at: https://www.rbht.nhs.uk/our-services/clinical_support/critical-care-and-anaesthesia/ecmo-and-severe-respiratory-failure/ecmo-referrals-and-transfer-pathway

Smith S, Scarth E. *Drugs in Anaesthesia and Intensive Care*, 5th edition. Oxford University Press, 2016. Nitric oxide.

5. B

The incidence of pulmonary embolism in pregnancy is common— between 1.4–4.2%. Anticoagulants should be started promptly and continued until pulmonary embolism (PE) is excluded. Diagnostic testing is required, but it should not delay treatment. IV unfractionated heparin is preferred in massive PE with cardiovascular compromise. At term, IV unfractionated heparin should also be considered over low-molecular-weight heparins (LMWH) as it is more easily manipulated around labour and delivery. Given that she feels well in herself and is afebrile, a diagnosis of infection or sepsis is less likely than a PE, but it would be prudent to observe closely and treat if indicated.

Further reading

RCOG. Thromboembolic Disease in Pregnancy and the Puerperium: Acute Management. Green-top Guideline No 37b, 2015. Available at: https://www.rcog.org.uk/media/wj2lpco5/gtg-37b-1.pdf

Smith S, Scarth E. *Drugs in Anaesthesia and Intensive Care*, 5th edition. Oxford University Press, 2016. Heparins.

6. C

This child has severe croup (laryngotracheobronchitis). It is important to keep the child as calm as possible, or his condition will deteriorate. Therefore, both A and E are incorrect. In mild versions of croup with minimal stridor and well-maintained oxygenation, it would be appropriate to give just oral dexamethasone or nebulized budesonide if the child can't tolerate oral medication and observe. However, in this case, he is demonstrating significant upper airway obstruction and so answer C is the most appropriate next action to take.

Further reading

Scarth E, Smith S. *Drugs in Anaesthesia and Intensive Care*, 5th edition. Oxford University Press, 2016. Adrenaline.

7. E

Data from the NAP6 audit demonstrates that antibiotics are the most common trigger for anaphylaxis and teicoplanin is 17-fold more likely than other antibiotics. Muscle relaxants and chlorhexidine are the next most common triggers. Bronchospasm was the presenting feature in 18% of cases. Hypotension was the most common presenting symptom seen in 47% of cases, and present at some point in all episodes. Suxamethonium anaphylaxis presents mostly with bronchospasm and is twice as likely a cause than other muscle relaxants. The onset is rapid for antibiotics and muscle relaxants but delayed with chlorhexidine. This is likely secondary to the mode of absorption being slower with topical or subcutaneous administration.

Further reading

RCOA. NAP6 Report: Anaesthesia, Surgery and Life-threatening Anaphylactic Reactions, 2018. Available at: https://www.nationalauditprojects.org.uk/NAP6Report

Smith S, Scarth E. *Drugs in Anaesthesia and Intensive Care*, 5th edition. Oxford University Press, 2016. Atracurium, Mivacurium, Rocuronium, Suxamethonium, Vecuronium.

Drugs affecting the gastrointestinal system

Multiple-Choice Questions

1. Regarding ondansetron

A Alteration of the dose is required in patients with renal impairment

B Alteration of the dose is required in patients with hepatic impairment

C It impairs gastric motility

D 60–65% is absorbed following oral administration

E It acts both centrally and peripherally

2. Regarding terlipressin/glypressin

A It is identical to endogenous human vasopressin

B Is a pro-drug

C Causes vasoconstriction via V2 receptors

D Vasodilates via vascular oxytocin-type receptors

E Has a longer half-life than desmopressin

3. Regarding the drug cyclizine

A Is a non-competitive H1 receptor antagonist

B Has anticholinergic activity at nicotinic receptors

C Has greater oral bioavailability than ondansetron

D Is metabolized in the liver by N-demethylation

E Can produce tachycardia and hypotension due to alpha-blockade

4. Regarding omeprazole

A Is a furan derivative

B Inhibits the activity of the gastric chief cell

C Has a smaller volume of distribution than ranitidine

D Is predominantly excreted unchanged by the kidney

E Is associated with a decreased incidence of ventilator-associated pneumonia

5. Regarding the drug domperidone

A An intravenous dose should be administered over 5 minutes

B Has high first-pass metabolism lowering oral bioavailability

C Decreases lower oesophageal tone while increasing gastric emptying

D Dose should be reduced in patients with renal impairment

E Is primarily excreted unchanged in the urine

6. Regarding the oral bioavailability of antiemetics

A Haloperidol bioavailability is less than 25%

B Ondansetron peak plasma concentration occurs between 1 to 2 hours

C Domperidone undergoes minimal first-pass metabolism

D Metoclopramide is variably first-pass conjugated to sulphate

E The bioavailability of cyclizine is 80%

7. Glycopyrronium

A Is a quaternary ammonium compound

B Its vagolytic effect lasts 20–30 minutes

C Is unable to cross the blood–brain barrier

D Reduces gastric volume by 90%

E Antisialagogue activity lasts up to 1-hour post IV administration

Single Best Answers

1. You are reviewing a 37-year-old female patient in the intensive care unit (ICU). She underwent an emergency laparotomy three days previously for management of a perforated duodenal ulcer. She has a background of chronic non-steroidal anti-inflammatory drug (NSAID) use. She was successfully extubated on day two and has significantly improved clinically. You are planning continued treatment. In addition to cessation of NSAID use, what represents optimal management of her peptic ulcer disease (PUD)?

A H_2 receptor antagonist (e.g. ranitidine) therapy for four weeks

B *Helicobacter pylori* eradication therapy (e.g. omeprazole, amoxicillin, and metronidazole)

C Offer *Helicobacter pylori* testing

D Omeprazole 10 mg once a day for eight weeks

E Omeprazole 40 mg once a day for four weeks

2. A five-year-old girl is scheduled for adenotonsillectomy surgery. She previously had severe postoperative vomiting following strabismus surgery. Which treatment strategy is most likely to reduce the risk of postoperative vomiting?

A Avoidance of nitrous oxide intraoperatively

B Cyclizine 0.5–1 mg/kg given at the end of surgery

C Dexamethasone 0.15 mg/kg IV and ondansetron 0.1 mg/kg IV, both given at the beginning of surgery

D Intraoperative intravenous fluid therapy of 10 ml/kg of compound sodium lactate

E Ondansetron 0.15 mg/kg IV given at the end of surgery

3. A 28-year-old male is about to be admitted to intensive care following a mixed overdose rendering him GCS 3/15, necessitating intubation and ventilation in the emergency department (ED) resus. He is suspected of having ingested paracetamol and pregabalin while intoxicated with alcohol. The timeframe of ingestion is unclear. He was last seen three hours prior to being found. Which plan represents optimal initial management?

A Await INR, VBG, U + E, FBC, and paracetamol level prior to deciding on treatment pathway

B Calculate the significance of ingestion (significant only if >75 mg/kg/24 hours)

C Delay 1 hour until collecting a 4-hour paracetamol level prior to deciding treatment pathway

D Give charcoal 50 g via a nasogastric tube

E Immediately commence acetylcysteine 150 mg/kg infusion over one hour

4. A 42-year-old female is admitted to ICU, having been intubated and ventilated for management of hypoxic respiratory failure with associated septic shock secondary to community-acquired pneumonia. On day two, she is clinically much improved, and is no longer requiring vasoactive support. However, she remains sedated, intubated, and ventilated. Which strategy represents optimal management in prophylaxis against gastric stress ulceration and gastrointestinal bleeding?

A Cessation of corticosteroid therapy

B Enteral nutrition via a nasogastric tube

C Only treat if risk factors arise

D Ranitidine 50 mg eight hourly IV

E Withhold prophylactic enoxaparin

5. A seven-year-old girl has undergone strabismus surgery. She is vomiting in the post-anaesthetic recovery unit, despite intraoperative administration of ondansetron 0.15 mg/kg. She had a prolonged overnight fast, and did not receive intravenous fluids. Which treatment option represents the best management for her established postoperative vomiting?

A Dexamethasone 0.15 mg/kg IV

B Droperidol 25 mcg/kg orally

C Further single dose of ondansetron 0.15 mg/kg IV

D Mandatory rehydration with oral fluids

E Metoclopramide 0.15 mg/kg IV

6. A 43-year male has been admitted to resus following an upper gastrointestinal haemorrhage. He has a background of alcohol abuse and is known to have oesophageal varices. Regarding the acute management of confirmed or suspected oesophageal variceal haemorrhage, which of the following represents optimal management?

A Antibiotic prophylaxis providing Gram-negative cover

B Omeprazole should be given as an 80 mg IV bolus followed by infusion

C Propranolol should be titrated from 40 mg twice daily to 80 mg twice daily

D Somatostatin 50 μg IV bolus followed by 25–50 μg/hr infusion

E Terlipressin 1 mg should be administered IV every 4–6 hours for 5 days

7. You are planning a presentation on enteral nutrition for multidisciplinary teaching within your local ICU. Which statement aligns best with the properties of gastrointestinal absorption?

A Facilitated diffusion is independent of a given concentration gradient

B Only non-ionized drugs may cross cell membranes

C The rate of diffusion across a given barrier is independent of the barrier surface area

D Weak acids have greater intestinal than gastric absorption

E Weak bases undergo greater gastric absorption than weak acids

ANSWERS

Multiple-Choice Questions

1. FTFFT

In patients with renal impairment, although systemic clearance is reduced resulting in an increase in the elimination half-life, this is not clinically significant, obviating dose reduction. Ondansetron undergoes significant hepatic metabolism by P450 enzymes. Although individual enzyme inhibition does not necessitate dose reduction, hepatic impairment prolongs the elimination half-life to 15–32 hours. It should be limited to 8 mg/24 days in hepatic impairment. Ondansetron does not impair gastric motility. Large bowel transit time is increased. It is completely and passively absorbed. Oral bioavailability is 60–65% following first-pass metabolism. Ondansetron is a highly selective 5HT3 antagonist, acting both centrally and peripherally. It blocks small intestine afferent vagal activity and 5HT activity in the area postrema.

Further reading

Smith S, Scarth E. *Drugs in Anaesthesia and Intensive Care*, 5th edition. Oxford University Press, 2016. Ondansetron.

2. FTFTF

Vasopressin is a naturally occurring nonapeptide prohormone synthesized in the paraventricular and supraoptic nuclei of the posterior hypothalamus. It is also available in three synthetic analogue forms: argipressin, terlipressin/glypressin, and desmopressin. Endogenous vasopressin (or ADH) and its synthetic analogues act via G-protein vasopressin receptors V1, V2, and V3, and also has affinity for oxytocin-type receptors.

Argipressin (8-arginine-vasopressin) is identical to endogenous human vasopressin. Terlipressin/glypressin is a pro-drug which is metabolized to form lysine-vasopressin upon cleavage of three glycyl residues. Vasoconstriction is mediated via V1 receptors. V2 receptors regulate water reabsorption at the distal renal tubule and collecting duct. They are also located at endothelial cells, allowing von Willebrand factor release. Activation of oxytocin-type receptors present in vascular smooth muscle results in the release of nitric oxide, leading to vasodilation. The half-life of terlipressin is 50–70 minutes, while that of desmopressin is 2–3 hours.

Further reading

Smith S, Scarth E. *Drugs in Anaesthesia and Intensive Care*, 5th edition. Oxford University Press, 2016. Vasopressin.

3. FFTTT

Cyclizine is a competitive H1 receptor antagonist, blocking central histamine receptors within the vomiting area of the chemoreceptor trigger zone. Anticholinergic activity is mediated by central muscarinic (M1, M2, and M3) blockade. The oral bioavailability of cyclizine is 80%, while that of ondansetron is 60–65%. Cyclizine is metabolized to norcyclizine by hepatic N-demethylation. This metabolite has little antihistamine activity. It has mild cardiovascular anticholinergic action. It can produce tachycardia and hypotension due to alpha-blockade.

Further reading

Smith S, Scarth E. *Drugs in Anaesthesia and Intensive Care*, 5th edition. Oxford University Press, 2016. Cyclizine.

4. FFTFF

Omeprazole is a benzimidazole derivative. Ranitidine is a furan derivative. It acts via a derivative that non-competitively, irreversibly inhibits the gastric parietal cell H-K-ATPase, thereby inhibiting the function of the parietal cell 'proton pump'. It is 95–96% protein bound resulting in a lesser volume of distribution of 0.3–0.4 L/kg, compared to the 1.2–1.8 L/kg Vd of ranitidine. It is completely metabolized via oxidation to a sulfone, reduction to a sulphide, and hydroxylation. 80% of an oral dose is excreted in the urine. As with other proton pump inhibitors, omeprazole is associated with ventilator-associated pneumonia.

Further reading

Smith S, Scarth E. *Drugs in Anaesthesia and Intensive Care*, 5th edition. Oxford University Press, 2016. Omeprazole.

5. FTFFF

Domperidone is butyrophenone derivative. There is no IV preparation available due to adverse cardiovascular effects associated with rapid intravenous administration. 90% of the drug is metabolized by hydroxylation and oxidative N-dealkylation. Oral bioavailability is 13–17% due to hepatic and gut wall metabolism. Domperidone increases lower oesophageal tone and increases the rate of gastric emptying. It appears to be more effective than metoclopramide in the treatment of established postoperative nausea and vomiting (PONV). Only 30% of domperidone is excreted in the urine. Its elimination half-life is 7.5 hours. It does not accumulate in renal impairment.

Further reading

Smith S, Scarth E. *Drugs in Anaesthesia and Intensive Care*, 5th edition. Oxford University Press, 2016. Domperidone.

6. FTFTT

Haloperidol has an oral bioavailability of 50–88%. This is affected by extensive hepatic metabolism, including reduction to an active metabolite.

Ondansetron reaches its peak plasma concentration of 30 ng/ml (following an 8 mg dose) in approximately 1.5 hours.

Domperidone undergoes significant first-pass metabolism. Oral bioavailability is 13–17%.

Metoclopramide is rapidly absorbed and is variably first-pass conjugated to sulphate. Its bioavailability ranges between 32–97%.

Cyclizine is well absorbed orally, with a bioavailability of 80%. Its peak plasma concentration reaches 70 ng/ml at approximately 2 hours.

Further reading

Smith S, Scarth E. *Drugs in Anaesthesia and Intensive Care*, 5th edition. Oxford University Press, 2016. Cyclizine, Domperidone, Haloperidol, Metoclopramide, Ondansetron.

7. **TFTTF**

Glycopyrronium is a quaternary ammonium compound in contrast to atropine, which is a tertiary amine. Its vagolytic activity last approximately 2–3 hours. The time course of action is better matched to neostigmine than atropine, leading to less late bradycardia. In view of its quaternary ammonium structure, glycopyrronium is unable to cross the blood–brain barrier. However, drowsiness and headache are recognized sequelae of its use. It reduces gastric volume by 90% at four hours after administration. It reduces lower oesophageal tone and decreases antral motility. Glycopyrronium has a powerful antisialagogue effect, five times more potent than atropine. This activity lasts for up to eight hours after intravenous or intramuscular administration.

Further reading

Smith S, Scarth E. *Drugs in Anaesthesia and Intensive Care*, 5th edition. Oxford University Press, 2016. Glycopyrronium bromide.

Single Best Answers

1. **C**

This patient most likely has PUD secondary to chronic NSAID use. Its cessation, where possible, is important for treatment. NICE guidance suggests full-dose proton pump inhibitor (PPI) or H_2 receptor antagonist therapy (H2RA) for eight weeks for patients who have been taking NSAIDs.

Omeprazole 10 mg once a day for eight weeks is considered a low dose/on-demand dose, and is inappropriate for initial treatment.

Offering *Helicobacter pylori* testing is the only option most in keeping with guidance. While the cause of her PUD is likely already known, were H. pylori to be suspected, testing should be offered prior to commencing eradication therapy if positive.

Omeprazole 40 mg once a day for four weeks represents 'double dose' PPI. It is not indicated for the initial treatment of PUD. Its time frame of four weeks in the context of prior NSAID use is also inappropriately short.

Further reading

NICE. Gastro-oesophageal Reflux Disease and Dyspepsia in Adults: Investigation and Management [CG184], 2014. Available at: https://www.nice.org.uk/guidance/cg184

2. C

Nitrous oxide may be used for anaesthesia in children without increasing the incidence of PONV. Intraoperative intravenous fluid therapy during paediatric anaesthesia may be associated with decreased PONV. However, these findings are based on weak evidence. Ondansetron and dexamethasone exhibit a synergistic effect in reducing the incidence of PONV in both paediatric and adult patients.

Further reading

Carr A, et al. *Guidelines on the Prevention of Post-operative Vomiting in Children*. Association of Paediatric Anaesthetists of Great Britain & Ireland, 2016.

Smith S, Scarth E. *Drugs in Anaesthesia and Intensive Care*, 5th edition. Oxford University Press, 2016. Dexamethasone, Ondansetron.

3. E

In any case of suspected paracetamol overdose where there is uncertainty regarding the timescale of ingestion +/− a polypharmacy overdose has occurred with or without alcohol, then there should be no delay in administering acetylcysteine. Acetylcysteine provides an alternative supply of glutathione which is depleted in paracetamol overdose.

Further reading

Smith S, Scarth E. *Drugs in Anaesthesia and Intensive Care*, 5th edition. Oxford University Press, 2016. Paracetamol.

Wallace CI, Dargan PI, Jones AL. Paracetamol overdose: an evidence based flowchart to guide management. *Emerg Med J*, 2002;19:202–205.

4. B

While the use of ranitidine and omeprazole is common in stress ulcer prophylaxis in ICU patients, the optimal management strategy is to try to establish enteral nutrition. Corticosteroid therapy is associated with the development of stress ulcers although it should only be discontinued if ongoing steroid treatment exposes more risk to the patient than stopping its administration. This decision should be made on an individual case-by-case basis. Administration of enoxaparin *per se* does not cause an increase in the incidence of stress ulcer, although its use should be reviewed if the patient exhibits signs consistent with a gastrointestinal (GI) bleed secondary to stress ulcer formation. It should also be noted that the use of omeprazole and ranitidine is associated with ventilator-associated pneumonia in critically ill patients.

Further reading

Smith S, Scarth E. *Drugs in Anaesthesia and Intensive Care*, 5th edition. Oxford University Press, 2016. Omeprazole, Ranitidine.

5. A

Dexamethasone has antiemetic properties and also exhibits a synergistic effect with ondansetron. Mandatory rehydration with oral fluids is unlikely to be successful while the patient has ongoing vomiting. Metoclopramide is associated with extrapyramidal side effects including akathisia and oculogyric crises in children and should be avoided.

Further reading

Smith S, Scarth E. *Drugs in Anaesthesia and Intensive Care*, 5th edition. Oxford University Press, 2016. Dexamethasone, Metoclopramide, Ondansetron.

6. A

There is good evidence for the administration of antibiotic prophylaxis resulting in a survival benefit.

Omeprazole is indicated for the management of upper gastrointestinal haemorrhage secondary to major peptic ulcer bleeding. There has been no bleeding or survival benefit demonstrated in variceal bleeding.

Propranolol is indicated for prophylaxis of variceal bleeding in portal hypertension. It should be titrated from 40 mg twice daily to 80 mg twice daily. It has no role in acute management.

A comparison of somatostatin, octreotide, and terlipressin has failed to show a bleeding or survival benefit. Octeotide should be administered by 50 μg IV bolus followed by 25–50 μg/hr infusion, while somatostatin should be administered by 250 mg IV bolus followed by 250 mg/hr infusion. Terlipressin 1 mg is licensed for administration every 4–6 hours for 72 hours. Five days of treatment has not been demonstrated to have a survival benefit.

Further reading

NICE. Gastrointestinal Bleeding: The Management of Acute Upper Gastrointestinal Bleeding. NICE Guideline, 2011.

NICE. Acute Upper Gastrointestinal Bleeding in Over 16s: Management [CG141], 2016. Available at: https://www.nice.org.uk/guidance/cg141

Smith S, Scarth E. *Drugs in Anaesthesia and Intensive Care*, 5th edition. Oxford University Press, 2016. Omeprazole, Propranolol, Vasopressin.

Tripathi D, et al. UK guidelines on the management of variceal haemorrhage in cirrhotic patients. *Gut*, 2015;64(11):1680–1704.

7. D

Facilitated diffusion requires a concentration gradient. Active transport can take place against a concentration gradient.

Only non-ionized drugs have sufficient lipid solubility so as to cross cell membrane lipids. Ionized, water-soluble drugs pass through aqueous channels. Both are forms of passive diffusion.

The rate of diffusion across a given barrier is greatly dependent on the barrier surface area. Along with concentration gradient, permeability coefficient, and barrier thickness, this parameter is defined within Fick's law of diffusion.

Although at a higher intestinal pH, weak acids will exist in a more ionized form, intestinal absorption is greater due to the larger surface area.

Weak acids undergo greater gastric absorption than weak bases. A weak acid (pKa 3–5) will exist in the non-ionized form in such acidic conditions (pH 1–3), aiding absorption. A weak base, however, will exist in its ionized, protonated form, reducing the rate of absorption.

Further reading

O'Shaughnessy K. Principles of clinical pharmacology and drug therapy. In Warrell D, Cox T, Firth J (eds) *Oxford Textbook of Medicine*, Vol 1, 5th edition. Oxford University Press, 2010. Chapter 10.1.

Drugs affecting the renal tract

Multiple-Choice Questions

1. You are asked to see an 87-year-old lady who has been booked on the emergency list for a laparotomy following a contrast CT showing bowel obstruction. Her past medical history includes hypertension, diabetes, and rheumatoid arthritis. Her regular medications are amlodipine, losartan, metformin, naproxen, and omeprazole. Her perioperative management should include withholding which medications?

A Naproxen

B Amlodipine

C Losartan

D Omeprazole

E Metformin

2. A 78-year-old man is in the post-anaesthesia care unit (PACU) following endovascular AAA repair. Pre-op bloods show Cr 137, Ur 10.6, eGFR 56. Current observations are respiratory rate 16 breaths per minute, oxygen saturations 96% on 4 L nasal O_2, heart rate 84 beats per minute, and blood pressure 92/54 mmHg (MAP 67). Which of the following could be used to reduce the risk of an acute kidney injury?

A Acetylcysteine

B 0.9% Saline infusion

C 1.24% Sodium bicarbonate infusion

D Theophylline

E Haemodialysis

3. Which of the following affect transmembrane sodium transport in the kidney?

A Amiloride

B Spironolactone

C Acetazolamide

D Mannitol

E Dopamine

4. Which of the following are effects of loop diuretics?

A Vasodilatation

B Metabolic acidosis

C Hypernatraemia

D Hypomagnesaemia

E Conductive hearing loss

5. Which of the following medications may need to be dose adjusted in a patient with a glomerular filtration rate of 15 ml/min?

A Erythromycin

B Gabapentin

C Heparin

D Lithium

E Phenytoin

6. Which of the following impair renal autoregulation?

A Bendroflumethiazide

B Ciclosporin

C Ketorolac

D Perindopril

E Sevoflurane

7. Which of the following cause renal failure by acute tubular necrosis?

A Clopidogrel

B Ciclosporin

C Gentamicin

D IV contrast

E Tacrolimus

Single Best Answers

1. A 68-year-old man is in cardiac intensive care, day two post-op on-pump coronary artery bypass grafting ×4. He has been oliguric over the past 24 hours with urine output 0.3 ml/kg/hr and his creatinine has risen from 84 micromol/L pre-op to 148 micromol/L. Other blood results: Urea 19, K 4.9, Na 132. How would you manage this situation?

A Six hourly bloods and ongoing review

B Continuous renal replacement therapy (CRRT)

C Dopamine

D Furosemide

E Intermittent haemodialysis (IHD)

2. A 72-year-old female with severe rheumatoid arthritis is on the ward being treated for cellulitis. She has developed haematuria and severe renal impairment. Crystals were seen on urine microscopy. Which of the following medications is the most likely cause?

A Ibuprofen

B Lansoprazole

C Methotrexate

D Simvastatin

E Vancomycin

3. A 68-year-old female presents to the emergency department with severe myalgia and weakness. Four months ago, she was diagnosed with hypertension and started taking amlodipine, aspirin, and simvastatin. In the emergency department (ED), her initial creatinine kinase (CK) is 6890 units/L. She is diagnosed with rhabdomyolysis secondary to statin use. The most important therapy to prevent acute kidney injury (AKI) in this situation is:

A Bicarbonate

B Dialysis

C Isotonic saline

D Loop diuretics

E Mannitol

4. What is the preferred inotrope for maintaining mean arterial pressure (MAP) during a live donor nephrectomy?

A Dobutamine

B Dopamine

C Metaraminol

D Noradrenaline

E Phenylephrine

5. You have anaesthetised a 36-year-old female for a laparoscopic-assisted nephrectomy. In addition to regular paracetamol, what postoperative analgesia would you prescribe?

A Diclofenac PR

B Epidural analgesia

C Fentanyl PCA

D Morphine PCA

E Oxycodone orally

6. You have been asked to anaesthetise a six-year-old boy with chronic renal failure on peritoneal dialysis for an appendicectomy. Which muscle relaxant would be the best choice in this case?

A Atracurium

B Cis-atracurium

C Rocuronium

D Suxamethonium

E Vecuronium

7. You are anaesthetising a 54-year-old man for a cadaveric renal transplant. Following a cautious induction, his blood pressure is 98/57 mmHg. His arterial blood gas (ABG), on FiO₂ 0.5, shows:

pH 7.38, pCO₂ 5.2, pO₂ 28, Na 134, K 5.1,
Lactate 1.4, HCO₃₋ 23, BXS −0.6, Hb 78.

You determine that he is intravascularly underfilled and would like to optimize his fluid status. Which fluid would be the best option to use?

A Hartmann's solution

B Hydroxyethyl starch

C Mannitol

D Normal saline

E Packed red blood cells

ANSWERS

Multiple-Choice Questions

1. TTTFT

This patient is at very high risk for developing a perioperative AKI. Non-steroidal anti-inflammatory drugs (NSAIDs), such as naproxen, carry a significant risk of nephrotoxicity, compounded when used in conjunction with angiotensin 2 receptor antagonists (A2RAs) and angiotensin-converting enzyme inhibitors (ACEis). They also increase the risk of contrast-induced nephropathy and therefore should be withheld. This patient is highly likely to need cardiovascular support perioperatively to maintain adequate perfusion pressure. It is therefore wise to withhold her antihypertensives until she regains her vascular tone. Any periods of hypotension and hypoperfusion will increase her risk of AKI. Metformin inhibits the metabolism of lactate and can cause lactic acidosis. This is particularly the case in patients with reduced renal function. Continuing omeprazole in this case will be beneficial for gastric protection.

Further reading

Scarth E, Smith S. *Drugs in Anaesthesia and Intensive Care*, 5th edition. Oxford University Press, 2016. A2RAs, ACE inhibitors, Metformin, Omeprazole.

2. FTTFF

Endovascular AAA repair requires a high IV contrast load and therefore has an associated risk of contrast-induced (CI) AKI. The only therapy that has been shown to reduce the risk of developing CI AKI is avoidance of hypovolaemia and adequate hydration with isotonic crystalloid. There is no proven benefit of sodium bicarbonate over saline despite theoretical benefits. There is insufficient evidence to suggest any benefit from any of the other options.

Further reading

Gross J, Prowle J. Perioperative acute kidney injury. *BJA Education*, 2015;15(4):213–218.

Scarth E, Smith S. *Drugs in Anaesthesia and Intensive Care*, 5th edition. Oxford University Press, 2016. Aminophylline, Paracetamol, Sodium bicarbonate.

3. TTFFT

Amiloride is a potassium-sparing diuretic which blocks Na^+ absorption in the distal convoluted tubule in exchange for H^+ or K^+. Spironolactone antagonizes the actions of aldosterone. It causes reduced sodium absorption by a reduction in the synthesis of Na^+ H^+ co-transporter, as well as Na^+ channels. Dopamine stimulation of the dopaminergic receptors at the proximal convoluted tubule inhibits the Na^+ $K^+ATPase$, thereby producing natriuresis and diuresis. Acetazolamide is a carbonic anhydrase inhibitor. It effectively blocks HCO_{3-} being reabsorbed in the proximal convoluted tubule, which leads to an increased concentration of Na^+ moving through to the distal convoluted tubule where the higher Na^+ load will lead to a greater K^+ secretion and water will follow. Mannitol is an osmotic diuretic, which exerts its effects on the tubule lumen by reducing the effective Na^+ concentration and thus reducing the reabsorptive gradient.

Further reading

Clarke P, Simpson K. Diuretics and renal tubular function. *BJA, CEPD Reviews*, 2001;1(4):99–103.

Scarth E, Smith S. *Drugs in Anaesthesia and Intensive Care*, 5th edition. Oxford University Press, 2016. Acetazolamide, Amiloride, Dopamine, Mannitol, Spironolactone.

4. TFFTF

Loop diuretics produce a diuresis by inhibiting the Na^+ K^+2Cl- co-transporter in the ascending loop of Henle, thereby increasing Na^+ and water delivery to the distal convoluted tubule. By blocking this transporter, the oxygen consumption in the loop of Henle is reduced to basal levels and this may have a protective effect from ischaemia in the critically unwell. When given to patients with pulmonary oedema, the symptom of breathlessness improves before diuresis has occurred because of vasodilatation and reduction of ventricular preload. Electrolytes are lost in the diuresis causing disturbances, including hypokalaemia, hyponatraemia, hypomagnesaemia, and metabolic alkalosis. Ototoxicity, if it occurs, is sensorineural.

Further reading

Clarke P, Simpson K. Diuretics and renal tubular function. *BJA, CEPD Reviews*, 2001;1(4):99–103.

Scarth E, Smith S. *Drugs in Anaesthesia and Intensive Care*, 5th edition. Oxford University Press, 2016. Acetazolamide, Amiloride, Bendroflumethiazide, Dopamine, Furosemide, Mannitol, Spironolactone.

5. TTFTF

Lithium has a very narrow therapeutic/toxic ratio and therefore serum concentrations must be monitored. It is highly sensitive to changes in sodium and fluid status. Lithium is removed by haemodialysis. Renal impairment has little effect on the pharmacokinetics of heparin and as such does not require dose adjustment. Renal dysfunction itself is however associated with coagulopathy and therefore caution is advised. Erythromycin is excreted renally and therefore the dose should be reduced in renal impairment. It is not removed by haemofiltration or dialysis and so the dose should remain halved for patients undergoing these therapies. Gabapentin is excreted unchanged in the urine. Clearance is proportional to creatinine clearance, and therefore the dose should be reduced accordingly. In this patient, the BNF (British National Formulary) recommends a starting dose of 300 mg on alternate days in three divided doses. Gabapentin is removed by haemodialysis.

Further reading

Scarth E, Smith S. *Drugs in Anaesthesia and Intensive Care*, 5th edition. Oxford University Press, 2016. Gabapentin, Heparins, Lithium, Macrolides, Phenytoin.

6. FTTTF

As renal perfusion pressure is reduced the kidney is usually able to maintain blood flow and glomerular filtration through autoregulation. The initial response is decreased afferent arteriolar tone by tubuloglomerular feedback and direct myogenic responses. At a later stage, reductions in renal perfusion pressure lead to renin being released which results in more angiotensin II. Angiotensin II stimulates a preferential increase in resistance at the efferent arteriole to maintain intraglomerular pressure and glomerular filtration rate (GFR). Angiotensin-converting enzyme inhibitors therefore clearly impair this autoregulatory process. COX-2 inhibition by NSAIDs reduces the effect of vasodilatory prostaglandins at the afferent arteriole and increases the vasoconstrictive response to angiotensin II at the efferent arteriole. Ciclosporin causes nephrotoxicity by impairing tubuloglomerular feedback mechanisms and thus autoregulation of renal blood flow. Bendroflumethiazide and sevoflurane have no effect on renal autoregulation.

Further reading

Scarth E, Smith S. *Drugs in Anaesthesia and Intensive Care*, 5th edition. Oxford University Press, 2016. ACE inhibitors, Bendroflumethiazide, Ketorolac, Sevoflurane.

7. FFTTF

Aminoglycosides cause acute tubular necrosis. Tubular epithelial cell damage leads to occlusion of the tubular lumen. IV contrast media cause direct tubular necrosis and renal ischaemia. Ciclosporin, clopidogrel, and tacrolimus cause renal failure by thrombotic microangiopathy.

Further reading

Scarth E, Smith S. *Drugs in Anaesthesia and Intensive Care*, 5th edition. Oxford University Press, 2016. Aminoglycosides, Clopidogrel.

Single Best Answers

1. B

Cardiopulmonary bypass is a well-recognized risk factor for AKI. According to the 2012 Kidney Disease Improving Global Outcomes (KDIGO) criteria, this patient has stage 3 AKI. Dopamine increases postoperative urine output, but does not improve outcome. Diuretics, such as furosemide, should be limited to managing fluid balance as hypovolaemia may worsen the AKI. There is increasing evidence that early initiation of renal replacement therapy (RRT) improves survival and renal function outcomes. In the UK continuous RRT is the predominant mode of delivery.

Further reading

Council of the Intensive Care Society. *Standards and Recommendations for the Provision of Renal Replacement Therapy on Intensive Care Units in the United Kingdom*. Council of the Intensive Care Society, 2009.

Gross J, Prowle J. Perioperative acute kidney injury. *BJA Education*, 2015;15(4):213–218.

Scarth E, Smith S. *Drugs in Anaesthesia and Intensive Care*, 5th edition. Oxford University Press, 2016. Dopamine, Furosemide.

Webb S, Allen J. Perioperative renal protection. *Cont Educ Anaesth Crit Care Pain*, 2008;8(5):176–180.

2. C

All of these drugs can cause AKI. However, only methotrexate has been associated with crystal formation. The risk of methotrexate-induced nephrotoxicity is increased with hypovolaemia and high plasma concentration of the drug. Treatment is directed at volume repletion, washout of the crystals from the tubules with a loop diuretic, and alkalization of the urine.

Further reading

Anders H, Mulay S. Crystal nephropathies: mechanisms of crystal-induced kidney injury. *Nat Rev Nephrol*, 2017;13:226–240.

Scarth E, Smith S. *Drugs in Anaesthesia and Intensive Care*, 5th edition. Oxford University Press, 2016. Ibuprofen.

3. C

Plasma CK levels correlate with the severity of muscle injury. CK >5000 units/L puts this patient at high risk of AKI. In addition to stopping statin therapy, the prevention of AKI in this case relies upon the correction of volume depletion and prevention of intratubular cast formation. Initially fluid resuscitation with isotonic saline at 1–2 L per hour is appropriate. Despite the potential benefits of a forced alkaline diuresis with bicarbonate, there is no clear evidence that it is more effective than saline. Mannitol administration is not of proven benefit and risks hypovolaemia and hypernatraemia. Loop diuretics are only indicated if volume overload is present. Dialysis may be required if AKI is established, but is not indicated purely for removal of myoglobin.

Further reading

Martinek A, Petejova N. Acute kidney injury due to rhabdomyolysis and renal replacement therapy: a critical review. *Crit Care*, 2014;18:224.

Scarth E, Smith S. *Drugs in Anaesthesia and Intensive Care*, 5th edition. Oxford University Press, 2016. Aspirin, Furosemide, Mannitol, Sodium bicarbonate, Statins.

4. B

Maintenance of perfusion pressure at or above preoperative levels is essential in a live donor nephrectomy. Patients are usually preloaded with IV fluid and a positive balance is maintained throughout. If an inotrope is required, dopamine is the most commonly used. There is no evidence that it provides renal protection, but at low doses (1–5 mcg/kg/min) it causes a marked decrease in renal vascular resistance, with a corresponding increase in renal blood flow. Also at low doses, beta-adrenergic effects predominate, leading to positive inotropy, increased automaticity, cardiac output, and coronary blood flow.

Further reading

O'Brien B, Koertzen M. Anaesthesia for living donor renal transplant nephrectomy. *Cont Educ Anaesth Crit Care Pain*, 2012;12(6):317–321.

Scarth E, Smith S. *Drugs in Anaesthesia and Intensive Care*, 5th edition. Oxford University Press, 2016. Dobutamine, Dopamine, Metaraminol, Noradrenaline, Phenylephrine.

5. C

A multimodal analgesic regimen is the gold standard. There are special considerations however in patients with, or at risk of, renal impairment. NSAIDs are generally avoided due to the risk of nephrotoxicity, however, they can provide good analgesia and less nausea and vomiting. They could be used in this scenario for up to five days as long as the patient maintains good hydration. Oral analgesia will be unreliable in the immediate postoperative period. Epidural analgesia is often avoided due to concerns regarding hypotension and underperfusion. A local anaesthetic infusion via a wound catheter would be a good addition to her analgesic regimen. Morphine is avoided due to the risk of accumulation of active metabolites and subsequent toxicity.

Further reading

O'Brien B, Koertzen M. Anaesthesia for living donor renal transplant nephrectomy. *Cont Educ Anaesth Crit Care Pain*, 2012;12(6):317–321.

Scarth E, Smith S. *Drugs in Anaesthesia and Intensive Care*, 5th edition. Oxford University Press, 2016. Diclofenac, Fentanyl, Oxycodone, Paracetamol.

6. C

A rapid or modified rapid sequence induction is required here. Suxamethonium should be avoided due to the risk of hyperkalaemia. With the availability of sugammadex, rocuronium is the best choice (N.B. in patients with *severe* renal impairment, the excretion of sugammadex and the 'sugammadex-neuromuscular blocker complex' is prolonged and caution is advised). Chronic kidney disease (CKD) will prolong the action of rocuronium and vecuronium and therefore a peripheral nerve stimulator must be used to monitor block. Atracurium and cis-atracurium are metabolized through Hoffman degradation and ester hydrolysis which is independent of renal function. This makes them ideal muscle relaxants to use in the CKD population, but not appropriate when a rapid sequence induction is required.

Further reading

Guruswamy V. Anaesthesia for children with renal disease. *BJA Education*, 2015;15(6):294–298.

Scarth E, Smith S. *Drugs in Anaesthesia and Intensive Care*, 5th edition. Oxford University Press, 2016. Atracurium, Cisatracurium, Sugammadex, Suxamethonium, Vecuronium.

7. A

Fluid loading to maintain cardiac output, optimize renal perfusion, and reduce blood viscosity may improve outcomes. Delivering liberal fluid administration at the beginning of surgery, while avoiding high total infusion volumes, is likely to be beneficial. Hartmann's is the solution of choice as a balanced crystalloid. Normal saline can be detrimental to postoperative acid-base balance and should therefore be avoided. Hydroxyethyl starch is associated with renal injury and must not be given, however, human albumin solution would be an acceptable alternative if a colloid were required. Mannitol is commonly used as an adjunct to fluid therapy in cadaveric renal transplant surgery, but is given as a 0.5 g/kg bolus at the time of clamp removal. Although this patient is anaemic, the Hb transfusion target in renal transplant is 70 g/L. Allogenic cytomegalovirus (CMV)-negative blood should be used with caution due to the risks associated with transfusion. Cell salvage should be used if there is any concern about high blood loss in these cases.

Further reading

Mayhew D, Ridgeway D, Hunter JM. Update on the intraoperative management of adult cadaveric renal transplantation. *BJA Education*, 2016;16(2):53–57.

Scarth E, Smith S. *Drugs in Anaesthesia and Intensive Care*, 5th edition. Oxford University Press, 2016. Hartmann's solution, Mannitol, Sodium chloride.

Drugs affecting the endocrine system

QUESTIONS

Multiple-Choice Questions

1. Regarding dexamethasone:

A It can be administered orally

B Gastrointestinal calcium absorption is reduced

C It induces sodium and water retention

D It is metabolized in the lungs

E Plasma half-life is 36–54 hours

2. Regarding metformin:

A It triggers insulin release from pancreatic ß-cells

B It inhibits intestinal disaccharidase, leading to a delay in absorption of monosaccharides

C It increases insulin receptor expression and tyrosine kinase activity

D It suppresses hepatic gluconeogenesis

E It activates peroxisome proliferator-activated receptor gamma (PPARɣ)

3. The following statements are true concerning glucagon:

A It is secreted by the ß-cells of the islets of Langerhans

B Its use is associated with nausea

C It is positively inotropic

D Glucagon can cause tachyarrhythmias

E Use may cause hypokalaemia

4. A 48-year-old female presents with confusion. She is clinically euvolaemic, euthyroid, and haemodynamically stable.

Investigations are as follows:

- Na 120 mmol/L
- K 4.6 mmol/L
- Creatinine 59 µmol/L
- Serum osmolality 260 mOsmol/kg
- Urinary osmolality 264 mOsmol/kg
- Urinary Na 40 mmol/L

Which of the following drugs could have resulted in this clinical picture?

A Lithium

B Carbamazepine

C Fluoxetine

D 3,4-methylenedioxymethamphetamine (MDMA)

E Bisoprolol

5. The onset of action of subcutaneously administered insulin can be affected by the following:

A Exercise

B Hypovolaemia

C The species of insulin used (e.g. porcine, bovine, or human)

D The choice of site

E The addition of zinc

6. Regarding levothyroxine:

A It acts by combining with a receptor in the cell nucleus to reduce DNA transcription

B The effects typically manifest within 1–2 hours

C It increases the rate and depth of respiration

D It is conjugated with glucuronide and sulphate

E Elimination half-life is 6–7 days

7. You are due to anaesthetise a patient who is taking dapagliflozin. Which of the following statements regarding this drug are correct?

A It enhances glucose secretion in the proximal convoluted tubules via sodium-glucose co-transporter 1 (SGLT-1)

B It requires endogenous insulin to be effective

C Its use may lead to a reduction in blood pressure

D It is less effective when used in patients with renal failure

E It should be omitted during starvation due to the risk of ketoacidosis

Single Best Answers

1. Which of the following best explains the mode of action of glibenclamide?

A It binds to the benzamido site on SUR1 receptor

B It is a dipeptidyl peptidase-4 (DPP-4) inhibitor

C It is a glucagon-like peptide 1(GLP-1) analogue

D It is an α -glucosidase inhibitor

E Receptor binding triggering pancreatic ß-cell membrane depolarization

2. A patient is scheduled for morning surgery who is usually pre-scribed 10 units of insulin detemir once daily at night. What, if any, adjustment should be made to the regimen prior to surgery?

A Admit the night before and start a variable rate insulin infusion

B No change is required

C Omit dose the night before

D Reduce dose to 5 units the night before surgery

E Reduce dose to 8 units the night before surgery

3. Which of the following steroid doses are equivalent when com-pared with 20 mg hydrocortisone?

A Betamethasone 0.1 mg (relative glucocorticoid potency)

B Dexamethasone 0.75 mg (relative glucocorticoid potency)

C Methylprednisolone 50 mg (relative glucocorticoid potency)

D Prednisolone 1mg (relative mineralocorticoid potency)

E Prednisolone 20 mg (relative glucocorticoid potency)

4. A 65-year-old gentleman presents with abdominal pain, diarrhoea, wheezing, and flushing.

Investigations include:

- Urine 5-hydroxyindoleacetic acid (5HIAA) 164 µmol/24 hr (reference range <50 µmol/24hrs)
- Urine normetanephrine 312 µmol/24hrs (reference range <900 µmol/24hrs)
- Urine dopamine 412 µmol/24hrs (reference range <700 µmol/24hrs)
- CT demonstrates an ascending colon mass.

Which medication should be instituted prior to proceeding with surgery?

A Fludrocortisone

B Methylprednisolone

C Octreotide

D Phenoxybenzamine

E Salbutamol inhalers

5. Which of the following best describes corticosteroids' mechanism of action?

A By binding to a cytosolic glucocorticoid receptor, which translocates to the nucleus

B By formation of a complex with nuclear receptors to modulate transcription

C By forming complexes with cytokines to reduce their activity

D By reducing sodium channel opening times

E Through directly binding a G-protein coupled receptor

6. You have anaesthetized a gentleman for resection of a phaeo-chromocytoma. Pharmacological management of hypertension was instituted several weeks prior to the operation. Intraoperative hypertension and tachycardia have been difficult to manage during tumour handling and you have needed to administer a number of different agents. All hypotensive agents have been discontinued for over an hour and you are concerned as the patient has catecholamine-resistant hypotension. Which medication is most likely to have contributed to this?

A Esmolol

B Glyceryl trinitrate

C Phenoxybenzamine

D Phentolamine

E Sodium nitroprusside

7. You have given a prophylactic five-unit intravenous bolus of oxy-tocin following uncomplicated lower segment caesarean section. Which clinical effect might you expect?

A A duration of action of 4–6 hours

B Increased lower oesophageal sphincter tone

C Increased urine output

D Onset of action after 90 seconds

E Prolongation of QT interval

ANSWERS

Multiple-Choice Questions

1. TTFFF

Dexamethasone is a synthetic glucocorticoid, used in anaesthesia mainly for its antiemetic effects. It is available as topical preparations, tablets, oral solution, and vials for injection. It is a potent glucocorticoid and so produces all the physiological effects:

- stimulation of and increased number of $\alpha 1$ and β adrenoreceptors resulting in positive myocardial contractility and vasoconstriction
- reduced inflammatory response by reducing the release of cytokines and tumour necrosis factor
- increased risk of peptic ulceration
- reduced gastrointestinal calcium uptake and increased renal excretion
- increased glomerular filtration rate and stimulated tubular secretion
- stimulated gluconeogenesis
- inhibition of peripheral utilization of glucose
- fat redistribution
- enhanced lipolysis
- reduced conversion of amino acids to proteins
- inhibition of endogenous corticosteroid release
- reduced fibroblast proliferation
- organ maturation in the foetus

Of note, dexamethasone has little mineralocorticoid activity and so does not cause sodium or water retention. It is up to 77% protein bound with high uptake after administration in the liver, kidney, and adrenal glands. It is metabolized slowly in the liver and excreted largely as unconjugated steroids in the urine. Plasma half-life is only 3.5–4.5 hours but the biological effects persist considerably longer with a biological half-life of 36–54 hours.

Further reading

Smith S, Scarth E. *Drugs in Anaesthesia and Intensive Care*, 5th edition. Oxford University Press, 2016. Dexamethasone.

2. FTTTF

Metformin is a dimethylbiguanide, and the only surviving member of the biguanide group (the other drugs resulted in a high rate of lactic acidosis and were withdrawn).

For metformin to be effective, there must be circulating insulin. There are a number of mechanisms of action but the main contribution to its effect is to stop glucose from rising through reduced hepatic gluconeogenesis. It is thought to reactivate hepatic adenosine monophosphate kinase (AMPK) and inhibit glucagon signalling, leading to a reduction in glycogenolysis and gluconeogenesis.

In addition, metformin increases insulin receptor expression and tyrosine kinase activity therefore increasing insulin sensitivity. There is an increase in glucose transport type 4 protein (GLUT-4) on skeletal muscle cell membrane enhancing insulin-stimulated glucose uptake and muscle glycogenesis. It also inhibits intestinal disaccharidase leading to a delay in the absorption of monosaccharides and a reduction in the rate of increase of blood glucose.

Thiazolidinediones (e.g. pioglitazone) activate peroxisome proliferator-activated receptor gamma (PPARγ) which forms a complex with retinoid X receptor and bound retinoic acid. The activated receptor locates a nucleotide sequence termed the 'peroxisome proliferator response element' altering a range of genes involved in insulin sensitivity, glucose, and lipid metabolism.

Further reading

Bailey CJ, Davies MJ. *Oxford Textbook of Endocrinology and Diabetes*, 2nd edition. Oxford University Press, 2011. Pharmacological therapy of hyperglycaemia in type 2 diabetes mellitus.

Stubbs DJ, Levy N, Dhatariya K. Diabetes medication pharmacology. *BJA Education*, 2017;17(6):198–207.

3. FTTFT

Glucagon is a polypeptide hormone secreted by the α-cells of the pancreatic islets of Langerhans. Among its indications include the treatment of hypoglycaemia, cardiogenic shock, and potentially in β-blocker and calcium channel blocker overdose. It acts via cell membrane receptors to activate adenylate cyclase through a G_s protein leading to increased intracellular cAMP and therefore calcium concentrations.

Onset of action is within 1 minute when administered intravenously and within 8–10 minutes when given intramuscularly or subcutaneously. It leads to marked inotropy and to a lesser degree chronotropy. It does not increase the chance of arrhythmias. It reduces gastrointestinal tone and inhibits gastric and pancreatic secretions.

Metabolic effects include:

- gluconeogenesis
- glycogenolysis
- lipolysis, increased free fatty acids, and ketogenesis
- increased amino acid uptake and proteolysis
- increased calcium uptake into myocardial cells
- hypokalaemia secondary to increased insulin secretion

Diarrhoea, nausea, and vomiting and allergic phenomena may complicate its use. The elimination half-life is 3–6 minutes.

Further reading

McEnvoy MD, Furse CM. *Advanced Perioperative Crisis Management*. Oxford University Press, 2017. Beta blocker/calcium channel blocker overdose.

Smith S, Scarth E. *Drugs in Anaesthesia and Intensive Care*, 5th edition. Oxford University Press, 2016. Glucagon.

4. FTTTF

This patient has the syndrome of inappropriate antidiuretic hormone (SIADH). Increased antidiuretic hormone (ADH) acts on G-protein vasopressin receptors leading to increased apical cell membrane aquaporin-2 in the distal renal tubule and collecting ducts increasing water reabsorption (via V2 receptors). SIADH is characterized by hyponatraemia (Na <135 mmol/L), euvolaemia, low serum osmolality (<270 mOsmol/kg), and concentrated urine (urinary Na >20 mmol/L, urinary osmolality >100 mOsmol/kg).

Causes of SIADH include:

- malignancy (e.g. carcinoma, thymoma, lymphoma, carcinoid)
- pulmonary (e.g. pneumonia, TB, sarcoidosis)
- intracranial (e.g. trauma, infection, subarachnoid haemorrhage, stroke, post-surgical)
- others (e.g. HIV, Guillan–Barré syndrome)

Drug causes include: carbamazepine (typically mild hyponatraemia, but in large doses can be severe), SSRIs, MAOIs, MDMA (ecstasy), oxytocin, and chemotherapeutic agents. Lithium causes nephrogenic diabetes insipidus (hypernatraemia, raised serum osmolality). Bisoprolol has not been associated with sodium disturbance.

The underlying cause should be identified and treated. Water intake should be restricted although rarely saline infusion is required. Rapid correction should be avoided due to the risk of central pontine myelinolysis. Demeclocycline induces a nephrogenic diabetes insipidus and can be used for treatment. Specific V2-receptor antagonists such as tolvaptan may also be used.

Further reading

Hirst C, Allahabadia A, Cosgrove J. The adult patient with hyponatraemia. *Cont Educ Anaesth Crit Care Pain*, 2015;15(5):248–252.

Pal A, et al. Disorders of the posterior pituitary gland. In Warrell DA, Cox TM, Firth JD (eds) *Oxford Textbook of Medicine*, 5th edition. Oxford University Press, 2010. Chapter 13.3.

Smith S, Scarth E. *Drugs in Anaesthesia and Intensive Care*, 5th edition. Oxford University Press, 2016. Vasopressin.

5. TTTTT

All of the general factors that affect the absorption of other drugs subcutaneously will affect that of insulin. Absorption is quicker in any scenario leading to greater local or general blood flow such as exercise, a hotter climate, and massaging of the site. Injection at the abdomen and arm gives the quickest onset while it is slower at the leg. In contrast, factors reducing regional blood flow such as hypovolaemia and cool climates will reduce absorption. These factors may have a noticeable effect on how quickly blood sugar rises and falls.

Human insulin is more lipophilic than porcine or bovine conferring a more rapid absorption and onset of action. There is an apparent increase in dose required of 20% when using bovine or porcine insulin when compared to human insulin.

In the circulation insulin is monomeric, but zinc formulations encourage insulin to form crystalline lattices. The size of these crystals can be altered by varying the pH which will affect the speed of absorption. Other additives include protamine.

Further reading

Dayan C, Williams G. Diabetes. In Warrell DA, Cox TM, Firth JD (eds) *Oxford Textbook of Medicine*, 5th edition. Oxford University Press, 2010. Chapter 13.11.1.

Smith S, Scarth E. *Drugs in Anaesthesia and Intensive Care*, 5th edition. Oxford University Press, 2016. Insulin.

6. FFTTT

Levothyroxine is a synthetically produced levoisomer of endogenous thyroxine (T_4). Triiodothyronine (T_3) is the active form of the hormone. Approximately 35% of levothyroxine is converted to T_3 peripherally (predominantly in the liver and kidney by deiodinases). T_3 acts by combining with a receptor in the target cell nucleus to activate DNA transcription, thereby increasing the rate of RNA synthesis and protein synthesis.

After administration, effects typically manifest within 24 hours although the peak effect is at 6–7 days. It leads to positive inotropy and chronotropy, an increase in systolic, and a fall in diastolic blood pressure and vasodilation. Due to an increase in the basal metabolic rate, there is an increase in respiratory rate and depth. Patients may exhibit a tremor, hyperreflexia, and an increase in gastrointestinal motility and appetite. Protein synthesis is enhanced as is lipolysis.

Levothyroxine is well absorbed orally and is highly protein bound with a very small V_D. It is conjugated with glucuronide and sulphate and excreted in the bile although 20–40% is excreted unchanged. The elimination half-life is 6–7 days.

A T_3 only formulation is available, with a lower corresponding dose, quicker onset, shorter time until peak effect and shorter elimination half-life.

Further reading

Smith S, Scarth E. *Drugs in Anaesthesia and Intensive Care*, 5th edition. Oxford University Press, 2016. Levothyroxine.

Wass J, Owen K. *Oxford Handbook of Endocrinology and Diabetes*, 3rd edition. Oxford University Press, 2014. Thyroid.

7. FFTTT

Dapagliflozin is SGLT-2 inhibitor, otherwise known as gliflozin. Other examples include canagliflozin and empagliflozin. In normal health, glucose filtered in the urine is almost entirely reabsorbed. Around 90% of glucose in the urine is actively reabsorbed by the SGLT-2 symporter in the proximal convoluted tubule and the remainder by SGLT-1. Gliflozins inhibit SGLT-2 glucose reabsorption resulting in loss in the urine of up to 70 g per day, resulting in reduced circulating glucose. This action does not require circulating insulin and is independent of insulin resistance, and results in a reduction in HbA1c of around 11mmol/mol. This effect is less pronounced in patients with severe renal impairment due to the reduced glomerular filtration of glucose. Use results in polyuria, reduction in systolic and diastolic blood pressure, and weight loss. Diabetic ketoacidosis has rarely been associated with their use and so it is recommended that they are omitted in fasting patients.

Further reading

Davey P, Sprigings D. *Diagnosis and Treatment in Internal Medicine*. Oxford University Press, 2018. Diabetes mellitus.

Stubbs DJ, Levy N, Dhatariya K. Diabetes medication pharmacology. *BJA Education*, 2017;17(6):198–207.

van Baar MJB, et al. SGLT2 Inhibitors in combination therapy: from mechanisms to clinical considerations in type 2 diabetes management. *Diabetes Care*, 2018;41(8):1543–1556.

Single Best Answers

1. E

Glibenclamide is a sulphonylurea. They bind to a specific sulphonylurea site on the sulphonylurea receptor 1 (SUR1) on pancreatic ß cells which is part of a transmembrane protein complex. This leads to the closure of a linked K_{ATP} channel, preventing potassium efflux, which causes membrane depolarization. This opens adjacent L-type calcium channels, causing calcium influx, thus activating calcium-sensitive signalling proteins which ultimately leads to increased insulin secretion.

Meglitinides (e.g. repaglinide) bind to a different (benzamido) site on the SUR1 receptor causing the same changes as sulphonylureas. They are more rapidly acting with a shorter duration of action.

GLP-1 is an incretin hormone produced by the L cells of the gastrointestinal (GI) tract in response to glucose. Its effects include enhancing insulin secretion, inhibiting glucagon secretion, reducing gastric emptying (slowing the rise in serum glucose), and promoting satiety. GLP-1 analogues (e.g. exenatide) must be given subcutaneously. GLP-1 is broken down by DPP-4. The DPP-4 inhibitors (otherwise known as gliptins) such as sitagliptin can be used to improve glycaemic control.

α -glucosidase inhibitors (e.g. acarbose) bind to the enzyme preventing the binding and cleavage of oligosaccharides into monosaccharides impeding carbohydrate digestion, and slowing serum glucose rise.

Further reading

Bailey CJ, Davies MJ. *Oxford Textbook of Endocrinology and Diabetes*, 2nd edition. Oxford University Press, 2011. Pharmacological therapy of hyperglycaemia in type 2 diabetes mellitus.

Smith S, Scarth E. *Drugs in Anaesthesia and Intensive Care*, 5th edition. Oxford University Press, 2016. Sulfonylureas.

Stubbs DJ, Levy N, Dhatariya K. Diabetes medication pharmacology. *BJA Education*, 2017;17(6):198–207.

2. E

The CPOC guidelines around use of long-acting insulins suggests for once daily long-acting insulin administered in the evening, the dose should be reduced by 20% regardless of whether surgery is in the morning or evening. If the long-acting insulin is normally taken in the morning, then a dose reduced by 20% may be given on the morning of surgery.

Insulin detemir is a long-acting insulin analogue. Other examples include glargine and degludec. Alterations in the insulin molecule prolong the duration of action. For instance, the action of detemir is delayed due to the addition of a fatty acyl chain that binds to plasma proteins like albumin. Glargine has two extra arginines extending the C-terminal of the B chain, leading to it precipitating under the skin due to the change in pH.

A feature of the long-acting insulin analogues is a 'peakless' profile with a long duration of action of between 18 and 36 hours. They are given either once or twice daily, often with pre-prandial short-acting insulin to cover mealtime peaks.

Further reading

Association of Anaesthetists of Great Britain and Ireland. Peri-operative management of the surgical patient with diabetes 2015. *Anaesthesia*, 2015;70:1427–1440.

Centre for Perioperative Care. Guideline for Perioperative Care for People with Diabetes Mellitus Undergoing Elective and Emergency Surgery. *CPOC*, 2021.

Dayan C, Williams G. Diabetes. In Warrell DA, Cox TM, Firth JD (eds) *Oxford Textbook of Medicine*, 5th edition. Oxford University Press, 2010. Chapter 13.11.1.

Stubbs DJ, Levy N, Dhatariya K. Diabetes medication pharmacology. *BJA Education*, 2017;17(6):198–207.

3. B

See Table 15.1. Hydrocortisone has equal mineralocorticoid and gluco-corticoid potency and has the shortest half-life of the available prepar-ations at 8 hours. Prednisolone and methylprednisolone are four and five times the glucocorticoid potency respectively, but both have relatively lower mineralocorticoid potency. Importantly both dexamethasone and betamethasone lack any mineralocorticoid activity and have among the longest half-lives. Fludrocortisone has the greatest relative mineralocor-ticoid potency.

Cortisol is produced by the adrenal gland at a rate of around 10–15 mg/day, but this increases significantly with stress. Awareness of the relative strengths of steroids is important peri-operatively to guide replacement in patients lacking the intrinsic response to stress because of disease or from hypothalamic-pituitary-adrenal axis suppression from long-term steroid use.

Glucocorticoid effects include maintaining circulatory tone, heightening mental awareness, gluconeogenesis, redistribution of body fat, enhanced lipolysis, and reduced amino acid to protein conversion. It produces pro-found anti-inflammatory effects. In contrast, mineralocorticoid action increases sodium reabsorption and potassium and hydrogen ion excre-tion and increases arteriolar tone via the renin-angiotensin-aldosterone system.

Further reading

Gupta A, Singh-Radcliff N. *Pharmacology in Anesthesia Practice*. Oxford University Press, 2013. Steroids.

McEvoy MD, Furse CM. *Advanced Perioperative Crisis Management*. Oxford University Press, 2017. Perioperative adrenal crisis.

Smith S, Scarth E. *Drugs in Anaesthesia and Intensive Care*, 5th edition. Oxford University Press, 2016. Prednisolone.

Table 15.1 Table of relative glucocorticoid and mineralocorticoid potencies of some common steroids

	Glucocorti-coid dose (mg)	Relative glucocorti-coid potency	Relative mineralo-corticoid potency	Plasma half-life (hrs)
Hydrocortisone	20	1	1	8
Prednisolone	5	4	0.8	16–36
Methylprednisolone	4	5	0.5	18–40
Dexamethasone	0.75	30	0	36–54
Betamethasone	0.6	25	0	36–54

4. C

This patient has carcinoid syndrome, as evidenced by his symptoms and raised 24-hour urine 5HIAA. The syndrome effects approximately 10% of patients with carcinoid tumours and is caused by tumour serotonin secretion. These neuroendocrine tumours most often occur in the GI tract but may also occur in the broncho-pulmonary system. Other symptoms that may occur include lacrimation and rhinorrhoea.

The precursor for serotonin is tryptophan. Serotonin is metabolized via monoamine oxidase (MAO) to 5HIAA which is then excreted in the urine. Somatostatin is a polypeptide hormone that inhibits tumour hormone release. It is also a potent inhibitor of growth hormone, insulin, and glucagon.

In addition to other standard preoperative planning for major surgery, patients should be assessed for the presence of right heart valvular disease. Due to the risk of perioperative uncontrolled hormone release, which may result in hypo- or hypertensive crises, a somatostatin analogue should be instituted.

Octreotide is a short-acting somatostatin analogue and is highly effective in improving symptoms. It may cause QT prolongation, bradycardia, conduction delay, abdominal cramping, and nausea. Further dosing of octreotide may be required preoperatively if symptoms remain uncontrolled.

Further reading

Powell B, Al Mukhtar A, Mills GH. Carcinoid: the disease and its implications for anaesthesia. *Cont Educ Anaesth Crit Care Pain*, 2011;11(1):9–13.

Strosberg JR. Diagnosis of Carcinoid Syndrome and Tumor Localization. UpToDate, 2018. Available at: https://www.uptodate.com/conte nts/diagnosis-of-the-carcinoid-syndrome-and-tumor-localization?sea rch=carcinoid&source=search_result&selectedTitle=1~150&usage_t ype=default&display_rank=1

Strosberg JR. Treatment of the Carcinoid Syndrome. UpToDate, 2018. Available at: https://www.uptodate.com/contents/treatment-of-the-carcinoid-syndrome?search=carcinoid%20syndrome&source=search_result&selectedTitle=1~150&usage_type=default&display_rank=1

Young WF. Clinical Presentation and Diagnosis of Pheochromocytoma. UpToDate, 2018. Available at: https://uptodate.com/contents/clini cal-presentation-and-diagnosis-of-pheochromocytoma

5. A

Corticosteroids diffuse across cell membranes to react with cytoplasmic receptors to form a complex which translocates to the nucleus. Here it binds to 'glucocorticoid response elements' to influence the expression of pro- and anti-inflammatory genes, stimulate protein synthesis, and in particular direct synthesis of lipocortins. Their actions are antiallergic, antitoxic, antishock, antipyretics, and immunosuppressive in action. They reduce the expression of a number of cytokines (including interleukin 1–3, 6, TNF-α, and γ-interferon) and inhibit T-cell and monocyte activation and migration. Very high doses may cause T-cell lysis. In addition, they act on specific receptors on the plasma membrane of the hypothalamic–pituitary–adrenal axis.

Further reading

Smith S, Scarth E. *Drugs in Anaesthesia and Intensive Care*, 5th edition. Oxford University Press, 2016. Prednisolone.

Torpey N, Moghal NE, Watson E, Talbot D. *Renal Transplantation (Oxford Specialist Handbooks)*. Oxford University Press, 2010. Immunosuppression.

6. C

See Table 15.2. α-blockade with either phenoxybenzamine or doxazosin is commenced at least 7–14 days preoperatively, followed by selective ß1-blockade aiming to minimize dramatic haemodynamic responses to stimulation and tumour handling.

Phenoxybenzamine covalently binds to α-adrenergic receptors producing irreversible blockade resulting in a decrease in peripheral vascular resistance and reflex tachycardia. Oral bioavailability is 20–30%; it is metabolized by deacetylation in the liver and is excreted in the urine and bile. Due to its half-life of 24 hours, it is usually discontinued 24–48 hours prior to surgery. All other agents mentioned above have short half-lives and duration of action and so phenoxybenzamine is the most likely culprit.

Catecholamine release may be induced by tumour handling intraoperatively leading to dangerous hypertension and tachyarrhythmias or bradycardias. Hypertensive crises should be managed with a vasodilator such as phentolamine, sodium nitroprusside, glyceryl trinitrate, or nicardipine. Tachycardia and tachyarrhythmias should be managed with ß-blockade using an agent such as esmolol.

Further reading

Connor D, Boumphrey S. Perioperative management of phaeochromocytoma. *BJA Education*, 2016;16(5):153–158.

Gupta A, Singh-Radcliff N. *Pharmacology in Anesthesia Practice*. Oxford University Press, 2013. Other antihypertensives.

Hardman JG, Hopkins PM, Stuys MMRF. *Oxford Textbook of Anaesthesia*. Oxford University Press, 2017. Cardiovascular drugs in anaesthetic practice.

Smith S, Scarth E. *Drugs in Anaesthesia and Intensive Care*, 5th edition. Oxford University Press, 2016. Phenoxybenzamine.

Table 15.2 Table of drugs used to manage hypertensive crises

	Mode of action	CVS effects	Onset	Duration	Half life
Phentol-amine	Reversible competitive α-adrenergic blockade. 3– 5 × more αl activity compared with α2	Reduced SVR, reflex tachycardia	1–10 mins	20–40 mins	10–15 mins
Sodium nitro-prusside	Stabilizes smooth muscle membrane preventing calcium influx by interacting with sulfhydryl groups	Decreases systemic blood pressure, compensatory tachycardia	30–120 seconds	2–5 mins	1–2 mins
Glyceryl trinitrate	Metabolized to nitric oxide which activates guanylate cyclase causing vascular smooth muscle relaxation	Venodilation at lower and arteriovenous dilation at higher doses, reflex tachycardia in health	1–5 mins	10–30 mins	1–3 mins
Esmolol	Competitive β-adrenoreceptors blockade, relative β1 selectivity	Fall in cardiac output of 20%, dose dependent fall in heart rate	1 min	12–20 mins	9.2 mins

7. E

Oxytocin is a naturally occurring polypeptide secreted by the posterior pituitary. It binds to specific receptors on the myometrium (of which there are a higher number during pregnancy), increasing the membrane excitability and leading to calcium influx. This stimulates uterine contractions.

When administered intravenously, oxytocin will act within 30 seconds with effects typically lasting for about 1 hour. An intramuscular dose will take 3–5 minutes to act and continue to act for 2–3 hours.

Hypotension is common (due to vascular smooth muscle relaxation) on bolus administration and often leads to reflex tachycardia. QT prolongation and T-wave flattening may occur. Oxytocin has no effect on the lower oesophageal sphincter tone. It is chemically similar to antidiuretic hormone and so promotes reduced urine output and water retention through a direct effect on the renal tubules. In high doses, this can lead to water intoxication and hyponatraemia.

Oxytocin is rapidly metabolized by hydrolysis in the liver and kidney with an elimination half-life of 1–7 minutes. Its use may cause reduced fasciculations and increased dose requirement with the administration of suxamethonium.

Further reading

Gupta A, Singh-Radcliff N. *Pharmacology in Anesthesia Practice*. Oxford University Press, 2013. Oxytocin.

Smith S, Scarth E. *Drugs in Anaesthesia and Intensive Care*, 5th edition. Oxford University Press, 2016. Oxytocin.

Drugs affecting the haematological and immune systems

QUESTIONS

Multiple-Choice Questions

1. Erythropoietin

A Can be administered orally

B Acts as a mitosis-stimulating factor

C Causes a dose-dependent increase in blood pressure

D Is a glycoprotein

E Is removed by haemodiafiltration

2. Regarding thrombolytic agents

A Include tranexamic acid

B Are derived from recombinant DNA technology

C Streptokinase acts directly on plasmin

D Are administered by bolus dose

E Once used, lead to the generation of antithrombotic antibodies

3. Rivaroxaban

A Is a benzamidine-based agent

B Indirectly inhibits factor Xa

C Affects platelet function

D Drug plasma levels may increase when administered with carbamazepine

E Drug plasma levels may decrease when administered with HIV protease inhibitors

4. Eptacog alfa (activated Factor VII)

A Is a vitamin K dependent glycoprotein

B Activates Factor X on the surface of platelets

C May cause disseminated intravascular coagulation (DIC)

D Can be used in conjunction with prothrombin complex

E Inhibitory antibody formation can occur following its use

5. Dabigatran

A Can be administered subcutaneously

B Is a non-reversible direct thrombin inhibitor

C Inhibits thrombin-induced platelet aggregation

D When co-administered with verapamil, may lead to reduced plasma drug levels of dabigatran

E Co-administration with St John's wort prolongs the duration of the effect of dabigatran

6. Fondaparinux

A Inhibits thrombin formation

B Binds to antithrombin III

C Affects platelet function

D Is used in the management of patients with Glanzmann's thrombasthenia

E Affects fibrinolytic activity

7. G-CSF (Filgrastim)

A Reduces the duration of neutropenia in patients receiving cytotoxic chemotherapy

B Is used in the mobilization of PBPCs (peripheral blood progenitor cells)

C Is indicated in the management of myelodysplastic syndrome

D May cause thrombocytosis

E Is rarely associated with musculoskeletal pain in patients receiving the drug

Single Best Answers

1. You are asked to review a 55-year-old woman in the emergency department who is having an ongoing upper gastrointestinal (GI) bleed. Her pulse is 140 bpm and her blood pressure is 98/56. She is known to be anticoagulated with warfarin for recurrent massive pulmonary embolisms (PEs). She is receiving IV fluids and packed red blood cells.

Regarding reversal of her warfarin, the next most appropriate action is:

A Give 4 units of fresh frozen plasma (FFP)

B Give prothrombin complex concentrate

C Give prothrombin complex concentrate and vitamin K

D Give recombinant factor VIIa (Eptacog alfa)

E Give vitamin K

2. A 28-year-old male is on your intensive care unit (ICU) following a staggered mixed overdose 12 hours ago. He was brought to the ICU due to a reduced level of consciousness, requiring intubation for airway protection. It is unclear as to the nature of all the agents he ingested but it does include dabigatran. A clotting screen demonstrates severe derangement in haemostasis. The ICU nurse comments that he is starting to bleed from his IV line sites.

Regarding reversing the effects of dabigatran, the next most appropriate action is:

A Administer 4 units of FFP

B Administer idarucizumab

C Administer prothrombin complex concentrate

D Initiate haemodialysis

E Insert a nasogastric tube and administer activated charcoal

3. You are asked to assess a 74-year-old man in resus. He was found collapsed in the street and currently has a Glasgow Coma Scale (GCS) of 9/15. A CT head scan without contrast has demonstrated a large subdural haematoma with midline shift. His case has been discussed with the regional neurosurgical unit, which has accepted the patient for neurosurgery. His only current medication is apixaban which he takes for secondary prevention of PEs as he is allergic to warfarin.

Regarding reversing the effects of apixaban, the next most appropriate action is:

A Administer 4 units of FFP

B Administer andexanet

C Administer ciraparantag

D Administer idarucizumab

E Administer prothrombin complex concentrate

4. A 62-year-old patient with diffuse large B-cell non-Hodgkin lymphoma is on ICU. He was admitted from the oncology day unit where he had been receiving intravenous therapeutic agents for his lymphoma treatment which included a red blood cell transfusion for symptomatic anaemia. He became erythematous, and developed bronchospasm and hypotension requiring admission for vasoactive support. He received IM adrenaline, IV hydrocortisone, and chlorphenamine at the time of the reaction. He is about to commence haemodiafiltration as he has severely impaired renal function with severe metabolic acidosis. His electrolytes are within normal limits.

The most likely diagnosis is:

A An acute transfusion reaction

B An anaphylactic reaction to a chemotherapy agent

C Cytokine-release syndrome

D Severe anaemia resulting in cardiac and renal failure

E Tumour lysis syndrome

5. You are asked to review a surgical patient on the ward. The patient is 22 years old and has a known diagnosis of melanoma for which he has been receiving treatment with curative intent. He has been receiving ipilimumab as part of his melanoma treatment. A PICC line is in place which appears clean and healthy. The only other significant finding in his past medical history is an open appendicectomy aged 12. Earlier today he was admitted to the ward via the emergency department with abdominal pain, bloody diarrhoea, nausea, and dehydration. There is a known norovirus outbreak in the local community and he is being barrier nursed in a side room. After his second cycle of treatment, he was admitted for 3 days with sepsis but no source was identified. A recent staging CT scan, performed 3 weeks ago, showed a reduction in tumour burden. His white blood cell count and C-reactive protein (CRP) are normal and he is apyrexial.

The most likely diagnosis is:

A An immune-related adverse event associated with ipilimumab

B Cytomegalovirus (CMV) colitis resulting from immunosuppressive treatment

C Malignancy associated bowel perforation

D Severe sepsis associated with immunosuppressive effects of cytotoxic chemotherapy

E Viral gastroenteritis

6. A 40-year-old patient is sedated and ventilated on ICU with severe ARDS. Fifty days ago he received an allogeneic stem cell transplant. He has been ventilated on ICU for 14 days and has had multiple diagnostic procedures to try to determine the cause of his respiratory failure. Chest radiography demonstrates perihilar interstitial/alveolar infiltrates with a 'ground-glass pattern' on high-resolution thoracic CT scanning. Bronchoalveolar lavage has failed to demonstrate causative microbes. He has been treated with high-dose co-trimoxazole. His peripheral blood film has been reported as normal.

The most likely diagnosis is:

A CMV pneumonitis as a result of immunosuppressive agents

B Interstitial pneumonitis secondary to immunochemotherapy agents

C *Pneumocystis jirovecii* pneumonia

D Pulmonary graft versus host disease (GvHD)

E Recurrence of original lymphoproliferative disease

7. You are asked to review a 45-year-old woman with a history of breast cancer who was admitted to ICU for respiratory support following an emergency admission via the emergency department with breathlessness and chest pain. She is currently receiving high-flow nasal oxygen therapy (60 L/min, FiO$_2$ 0.8). Her chest X-ray is consistent with pulmonary oedema. Prior to transfer to ICU she underwent a percutaneous coronary angiogram which demonstrated clear coronary vessels but a reduced LV ejection fraction. She is now complaining of pain in her right foot and leg. A haemostatic closure device over her right femoral artery has already been removed with no improvement in her symptoms. Her right pedal pulses are absent on doppler examination. Her breast cancer therapy was multimodal and included bevacizumab and paclitaxel.

The most likely *unifying* diagnosis is:

A Adverse vascular events secondary to bevacizumab

B Adverse vascular events secondary to paclitaxel

C Antiphospholipid syndrome

D Disseminated tumour emboli

E Malignancy associated vasculitis

ANSWERS

Multiple-Choice Questions

1. FTTTF

Erythropoietin is a glycoprotein used in the treatment of anaemia and is administered either subcutaneously (for preference) or intravenously. Erythropoiesis results from its activity as a mitosis-stimulating factor and differentiation hormone. In addition to erythropoiesis, it will also increase the platelet count but does not lead to thrombocytosis. A dose-dependent increase in blood pressure does occur with this agent. Erythropoietin is not removed by haemodiafiltration.

Further reading

Smith S, Scarth E. *Drugs in Anaesthesia and Intensive Care*, 5th edition. Oxford University Press, 2016. Erythropoietin.

2. FFFFF

Tranexamic acid exhibits antifibrinolytic activity and is not a thrombolytic agent. The thrombolytic agent, streptokinase, is derived from beta haemolytic streptococci of Lancefield Group C. However, other thrombolytic agents are produced using recombinant DNA technology. Streptokinase acts indirectly on plasmin. Thrombolytic agents may be administered by bolus dose or intravenous infusion depending on the specific agent being used and the clinical regimen. Only streptokinase administration leads to the generation of antistreptokinase antibodies.

Further reading

Smith S, Scarth E. *Drugs in Anaesthesia and Intensive Care*, 5th edition. Oxford University Press, 2016. Thrombolytics.

3. FFFFF

Rivaroxaban is an oxazolidinone derivative. It directly inhibits factor Xa in a dose-dependent manner, leading to interruption of intrinsic and extrinsic coagulation pathways, but has no effect on thrombin or platelet function. A proportion of the drug undergoes oxidative degradation and hydrolysis via cytochrome P450 3A4. Other cytochrome subenzymes and non-cytochromic mechanisms are also involved. Excretion is 50% renal, 50% faecal. Patients receiving CYP450 3A4 inducers, such as carbamazepine, will lead to reduced drug plasma levels of rivaroxaban. Likewise, the presence of a CYP450 3A4 inhibitor, such as HIV protease inhibitor, results in increased rivaroxaban plasma levels.

Further reading

Smith S, Scarth E. *Drugs in Anaesthesia and Intensive Care*, 5th edition. Oxford University Press, 2016. Rivaroxaban.

4. TTTFT

Activated factor VII is produced using recombinant DNA technology and is a vitamin K-dependent glycoprotein. The agent binds to tissue factor, resulting in the activation of factors IX and X, leading to thrombin production. Eptacog alfa also activates factor X on the surface of platelets, independently of tissue factor. Use of the drug may lead to the development of thrombus or DIC, in situations where there is increased tissue factor expression. The use of prothrombin complex with eptacog alfa is not recommended due to the increased risk of thrombotic events. Inhibitory antibody formation may occur in patients with factor VII deficiency.

Further reading

Smith S, Scarth E. *Drugs in Anaesthesia and Intensive Care*, 5th edition. Oxford University Press, 2016. Eptacog alfa.

5. FFTFF

Dabigatran is presented as an oral preparation in the form of a pro-drug, dabigatran etexilate. Hydrolysis of the pro-drug by plasma and hepatic esterases produces dabigatran, which is a competitive, reversible direct thrombin inhibitor preventing cleavage of fibrinogen to fibrin. Dabigatran also inhibits thrombin-induced platelet aggregation. The duration of drug exposure is increased when dabigatran is administered to patients receiving amiodarone and dose limitation is advised. The nature of this interaction is unknown, however, amiodarone is an inhibitor of the efflux transporter P-glycoprotein, of which dabigatran is a substrate. Verapamil is an inhibitor of P-glycoprotein, therefore co-administration would lead to an *increased* plasma drug level of dabigatran. St John's wort (P-glycoprotein inducer) would be expected to reduce the duration of effect of dabigatran.

Further reading

Smith S, Scarth E. *Drugs in Anaesthesia and Intensive Care*, 5th edition. Oxford University Press, 2016. Dabigatran.

6. TTFFF

Fondaparinux is a synthetic and specific inhibitor of activated Xa, mediated by antithrombin III. It selectively binds antithrombin III, potentiating 300-fold the neutralization of factor Xa, thereby inhibiting thrombin formation and thrombus generation. The drug is used in the treatment of acute PE/DVT and can also be used in the prophylaxis of DVTs. The drug has no effect on platelet function. Management of Glanzmann's thrombasthenia would require the use of an agent such as eptacog alfa. Fondaparinux has no effect on fibrinolytic activity or bleeding time.

Further reading

Smith S, Scarth E. *Drugs in Anaesthesia and Intensive Care*, 5th edition. Oxford University Press, 2016. Fondaparinux.

7. TTFFF

G-CSF (granulocyte colony-stimulating factor) is used in the management of patients receiving cytotoxic chemotherapy, to reduce the duration of neutropenia. It is also used for the mobilization of PBPCs in patients who will subsequently receive autologous PBPC transplantation. G-CSF is not indicated in the management of myelodysplastic syndrome. Thrombocytopaenia, rather than thrombocytosis, occurs in at least 10% of patients. Musculoskeletal pain is a commonly occurring side effect.

Further reading

Datapharm. Accofil 48 MU/0.5 ml Solution for Injection or Infusion in Pre-filled Syringe, June 2019. Available at: https://www.medicines. org.uk/emc/product/3383/smpc

Single Best Answers

1. C

The reversal of an anticoagulation agent depends on the degree of bleeding. In this case, this is a life-threatening upper GI haemorrhage. Prothrombin complex concentrate is indicated for the reversal of warfarin, however, administration in isolation should be avoided as the half-life is approximately six hours. The addition of vitamin K will help maintain haemostasis. Vitamin K alone would not work quickly enough to antagonize the effects of warfarin. Recombinant factor VIIa would only be considered if all other measures had failed and after discussion with a haematologist. Fresh frozen plasma is not recommended for warfarin reversal.

Further reading

McIlmoyle K, Tran H. Perioperative management of oral anticoagulation *BJA Education*, 2018;18(9):259–264.

Smith S, Scarth E. *Drugs in Anaesthesia and Intensive Care*, 5th edition. Oxford University Press, 2016. Prothrombin complex.

2. B

Dabigatran is a direct oral anticoagulant which reversibly inhibits thrombin. Activated charcoal is only indicated if ingestion has occurred within three hours of presentation to hospital. FFP is not indicated for the reversal of dabigatran. Idarucizumab is a monoclonal antibody fragment that binds to dabigatran with 350 times the affinity of dabigatran to thrombin, thereby preventing dabigatran from exerting its anticoagulant effect. If available, this agent should be used first line in this situation. Administration of prothrombin complex concentrate would be considered a second-line therapy. Haemodialysis is an option for clearing circulating dabigatran, but this will take time to be established and is associated with additional risk.

Further reading

McIlmoyle K, Tran H. Perioperative management of oral anticoagulation *BJA Education*, 2018;18(9):259–264.

Smith S, Scarth E. *Drugs in Anaesthesia and Intensive Care*, 5th edition. Oxford University Press, 2016. Dabigatran.

3. **B**

Apixaban is a factor Xa inhibitor. Administration of plasma is not recommended for its reversal. Idarucizumab is only licensed for use in the reversal of dabigatran. Ciraparantag is an investigational agent that is being developed as a 'universal antidote' to direct acting oral anticoagulation agents, fondaparinux, heparins, and low molecular weight heparins. It does not currently have a licence. Andexanet is modified recombinant factor Xa and as such binds to factor Xa inhibitors resulting in the reversal of their anticoagulant effect. Prothrombin complex concentrate could be used if andexanet was not available.

Further reading

McIlmoyle K, Tran H. Perioperative management of oral anticoagulation *BJA Education*, 2018;18(9):259–264.

Smith S, Scarth E. *Drugs in Anaesthesia and Intensive Care*, 5th edition. Oxford University Press, 2016. Prothrombin complex.

4. **C**

While an anaphylactic reaction to chemotherapy is possible, the appropriate emergency management steps were undertaken and it would be usual for these to limit such a reaction. Severe renal impairment is not a typical feature of anaphylaxis. Tumour lysis syndrome (TLS) is usually associated with rapidly dividing tumours (such as Burkitt's lymphoma and acute lymphoblastic leukaemia) that are chemo-responsive resulting in rapid tumour cell death. The typical features of TLS include hyperuricaemia, hyperphosphataemia, hyperkalaemia, and hypocalcaemia which are not seen in this case. An acute transfusion reaction is possible but unlikely. Cytokine-release syndrome (CRS) is a more likely diagnosis, especially given that the patient is receiving 'intravenous therapeutic agents' (N.B. not *just* cytotoxic chemotherapy agents) for the treatment of B-cell lymphoma of which the monoclonal antibody rituximab is known to cause CRS. Severe anaemia would take time to result in significant end-organ pathology and the clinical features fit more with an acute event.

Further reading

Kroschinsky F, et al. New drugs, new toxicities: severe side effects of modern targeted and immunotherapy of cancer and their management. *Crit Care*, 2017;21:89.

Smith S, Scarth E. *Drugs in Anaesthesia and Intensive Care*, 5th edition. Oxford University Press, 2016. Allopurinol.

5. A

Viral gastroenteritis could present with this constellation of symptoms but bloody diarrhoea is not a typical feature. Bowel perforation associated with his underlying malignancy seems unlikely, given the reduction in tumour burden and suggested response to therapy. CMV colitis can cause these symptoms in immunocompromised individuals but patients tend to be older and the clinical picture is not typical of an infectious process. An immune-related adverse event associated with his melanoma treatment should be seriously considered, especially if he has received a 'checkpoint inhibitor' such as ipilimumab or nivolumab. These agents are designed to improve the immune system's innate function to target and destroy tumour cells. The net result is an inhibitor of the inhibitory components of the immune system but this can lead to an overwhelming inflammatory response. Diarrhoea and enterocolitis are complications of ipilimumab therapy and there should be a high index of suspicion of perforation, so urgent assessment and management are needed in these cases.

Further reading

Kroschinsky F, et al. New drugs, new toxicities: severe side effects of modern targeted and immunotherapy of cancer and their management. *Crit Care*, 2017;21:89.

6. B

CMV pneumonitis and P. jirovecii are possible diagnoses but are unlikely given the failure to elicit any positive microbiological evidence of infection. GvHD commonly occurs in patients receiving stem cell transplants but pulmonary involvement typically occurs after 100 days. Recurrence of his original disease process is possible but seems unlikely as there is no other evidence suggestive of relapse. He will have been exposed to numerous agents during his initial treatment to reach remission, together with agents in the condition regimen pre-transplant, that would be implicated in drug-induced pulmonary pneumonitis. The incidence of non-infectious, drug-induced pneumonitis has been recorded as being as high as 15% in these patients.

Further reading

Kroschinsky F, et al. New drugs, new toxicities: severe side effects of modern targeted and immunotherapy of cancer and their management. *Crit Care*, 2017;21:89.

7. A

Antiphospholipid syndrome can be present with hypoxaemia (secondary to multiple PEs) and peripheral vascular occlusion, but pulmonary oedema is not a typical feature. Malignancy-associated vasculitis is rare in breast cancer. Bevacizumab is a monoclonal antibody that has antiangiogenetic effects. These are utilized to impair tumour cell proliferation by interrupting neoangiogenesis. However, these agents are also associated with adverse vascular events including arterial hypertension, congestive heart failure, and arterial thromboembolism (in this case, exacerbated by the percutaneous procedure the patient underwent). Paclitaxel is used in the treatment of breast cancer but does not have vascular side effects. Disseminated tumour emboli are very unlikely in the clinical context.

Further reading

Kroschinsky F, et al. New drugs, new toxicities: severe side effects of modern targeted and immunotherapy of cancer and their management. *Crit Care*, 2017;21:89.

Drugs in overdose

QUESTIONS

Multiple-Choice Questions

1. The following agents produce predominantly hallucinogenic effects:

A Amphetamines

B Gamma-hydroxybutyrate

C Lysergic acid diethylamide

D Synthetic cannabinoid receptor agonists

E Synthetic cathinones

2. The following agents are associated with hyperthermia:

A Belladonna alkaloids

B Gamma-hydroxybutyrate

C Lysergic acid diethylamide

D Muscarinic mushrooms

E Synthetic cathinones

3. Ingestion of the following agents may lead to mydriasis:

A Desomorphine 'Krokodil'

B Lysergic acid diethylamide

C Muscarinic mushrooms

D Phencyclidine derivatives

E Synthetic cathinones

4. Regarding lysergic acid diethylamide:

A   The agent is a semisynthetic ergoline drug

B   Has a half-life of approximately eight hours

C   When administered orally, clinical effects are seen within five minutes of ingestion

D   Synaesthesia occurs rarely

E   Can be detected in a urinary drug screen

5. The following agents can be detected in the urine

A   Buprenorphine

B   Cannabinoids

C   Cathinones

D   Methadone

E   Synthetic cannabinoid receptor antagonists

6. Features associated with acute cathinone toxicity include:

A   Central nervous system (CNS) depression

B   Hypotension

C   Miosis

D   Muscle weakness

E   Tachypnoea

7. Agents that are associated with the 'stimulant syndrome' include:

A   *Belladonna* genera

B   'Ecstasy'

C   Lysergic acid diethylamide

D   Mephedrone

E   'Spice'

Single Best Answers

1. You are asked to review a 40-year-old male in the emergency department (ED). He was initially found by a member of the public acting in a strange way but shortly after arrival by ambulance, he became extremely agitated. On your arrival to assess him he is being restrained by four security staff having assaulted a member of the ED nursing staff. No observations are possible but IV access was established by the ambulance crew and remains patent. He has received a total of 5 mg of midazolam intravenously from the ED staff with minimal effect. He has stigmata of IV drug use and scarring consistent with self-harming. He is known to the ED staff as a frequent attendee with drug-related complications. The ambulance crew recovered a bottle labelled 'bath salts' found close to the patient.

The next most appropriate action is:

A Insert a urinary catheter for urgent urinary drug testing

B Obtain a collateral history

C Perform an urgent CT head scan

D Rapidly review the patient with a view to further sedation including intubation and ventilation

E Take blood for urgent toxicology

2. You are asked to review a 37-year-old female patient who is sedated and ventilated on the intensive care unit (ICU). She was initially admitted to hospital with abdominal pain, vomiting, and watery diarrhoea, following ingesting 'food that had been foraged in woodland'. Thirty-six hours following her presentation to hospital she was admitted to ICU following a seizure on the ward. Since her transfer to ICU, she has developed acute hepatic impairment and acute renal failure.

Which of the following is the most likely causative agent that the patient has ingested?

A *Amanita* species

B *Coprinus* species

C *Gyromitra* species

D *Orellanine* species

E *Psilocybe* species ('magic' mushrooms)

3. A patient is known to have ingested an 'unknown illicit drug'. The following clinical features are present in this patient: mydriasis, hypertension, seizure activity, and hyper-reflexia.

Which of the following agents is most likely to have been ingested?

A Anticholinergic agent

B Cholinergic agent

C Hallucinogenic agent

D Opioid agent

E Sympathomimetic agent

4. You are asked to urgently attend the ED where a number of adult males have been brought to hospital following a public order disturbance. They describe having experienced the following: breathlessness, cough, wheezing, lacrimation, and rhinorrhoea.

What is the most likely agent they have been exposed to?

A Ammonia

B Chloroacetophenone

C Chlorobenzylidenemalononitrile

D Phosgene

E Sulphuric acid

5. A usually fit and well 27-year-old female is brought to the ED having been found collapsed outside a night club with a reduced Glasgow Coma Scale (GCS) following a seizure and evidence of vomiting. She was intubated for airway protection by a pre-hospital team and is currently sedated with a propofol infusion and is mechanically ventilated. She has a temperature of 39.9°C and is tachycardic and hypertensive.

Which of the following diagnoses is most likely?

A Amphetamine ingestion

B Heat stroke secondary to ingestion of ecstasy

C Malignant hyperpyrexia secondary to muscle relaxant use

D Malignant neuroleptic syndrome

E Phaeochromocytoma and non-compliance with antihypertensive treatment

6. You are part of a major incident response at your local hospital following an explosion at a concert venue. There are possible reports of an improvised device being detonated at the scene.

Which of the following is the most rapid form of detection?

A Chemical detector paper

B Fourier transform infrared spectroscopy

C Gas chromatography mass spectrometry

D Raman spectrometer

E Signs and symptoms of victims

7. A 64-year-old man who works in the nuclear industry is an inpatient on ICU having been transferred from the haematology ward. He initially presented to hospital with severe vomiting of unknown aetiology followed by the development of pancytopenia and neutropenic sepsis. In recent days he has begun to develop alopecia. Potential ingestion of an alpha radiation emitter has been postulated as a possible cause.

Which of the following alpha sources is considered to be the most dangerous?

A ^{241}Americium

B ^{239}Plutonium

C ^{210}Polonium

D ^{232}Thorium

E ^{235}Uranium

ANSWERS

Multiple-Choice Questions

1. FFTTF

While it is possible for all of these agents to cause hallucinations, it is only a *predominant* feature with synthetic cannabinoid receptor agonists (SCRAs) and lysergic acid diethylamide (LSD). Sympathetic stimulation occurs with cathinone and amphetamine use with hallucinations only occurring in more severe cases. Gamma-hydroxybutyrate has sedative-hypnotic activity. SCRAs are not detected by routine drug screens and include 'spice'. LSD is a potent hallucinogen.

Further reading

Dignam G, Bigham C. Novel psychoactive substances: a practical approach to dealing with toxicity from legal highs. *BJA Education*, 2017;17(5):172–177.

2. TFTFT

Agents that are stimulatory in nature are often associated with a raised temperature. In some cases, this can result in extreme hyperthermia. Muscarinic mushrooms are not associated with hyperthermia and gamma-hydroxybutyric acid (GHB) is associated with *hypo*thermia.

Further reading

Dignam G, Bigham C. Novel psychoactive substances: a practical approach to dealing with toxicity from legal highs. *BJA Education*, 2017;17(5):172–177.

3. FTFTT

Muscarinic mushroom ingestion results in a cholinergic-mediated toxidrome of confusion, coma, seizure activity, miosis, bradycardia, bronchoconstriction, and lacrimation. Desomorphine 'Krokodil' is a synthetic opioid and as such, ingestion results in opioid-related effects including CNS depression, miosis, bradycardia, respiratory depression, and decreased gastric motility.

Further reading

Dignam G, Bigham C. Novel psychoactive substances: a practical approach to dealing with toxicity from legal highs. *BJA Education*, 2017;17(5):172–177.

4. TFFTT

LSD is a semisynthetic ergoline drug, meaning it has a structural skeleton of the alkaloid ergoline. The drug undergoes hepatic metabolism via the cytochrome P450 enzyme system. It has a half-life of approximately 2.5 hours and when administered orally, clinical effects are seen within 30 minutes of ingestion. Synaesthesia is the development of cross-sensory perception when, for example, auditory stimulation results in an involuntary change in visual perception. This is a recognized but overall fairly rare occurrence with LSD ingestion.

Further reading

Bateman D, et al. *Oxford Desk Reference: Toxicology*. Oxford University Press, 2014.

5. TTFTF

Routine urinary drug testing only detects a limited number of illicit drugs. However, it is always valuable to take serum and urine samples to be stored by the chemical pathology lab in case more specific testing may be required either locally, or at a poisons centre. SCRAs are not detected in routine urinary screening, hence their attractiveness to be used in individuals who may undergo routine testing. Both naturally occurring cathinones, such as 'Khat', and synthetic agents, such as mephedrone, are not routinely detectable.

Further reading

Bateman D, et al. *Oxford Desk Reference: Toxicology*. Oxford University Press, 2014.

Smith S, Scarth E. *Drugs in Anaesthesia and Intensive Care*, 5th edition. Oxford University Press, 2016. Buprenorphine.

6. FFFFT

Cathinone toxicity results in sympathomimetic toxidrome. Common features include agitation, rigidity, seizures, mydriasis, hypertension, tachypnoea, hyperthermia, rhabdomyolysis, and hyponatraemia. Toxicity is more likely when synthetic cathinones have been ingested compared with naturally occurring substances such as Khat.

Further reading

Dignam G, Bigham C. Novel psychoactive substances: a practical approach to dealing with toxicity from legal highs. *BJA Education*, 2017;17(5):172–177.

7. TTFTT

Common features of the stimulant syndrome include CNS excitation, sweating, dilated pupils, tachycardia, hypertension, bruxism (teeth grinding), hypertonia, and hyper-reflexia. All of the listed agents may result in some or all of these symptoms/signs except LSD which has more hallucinogenic properties. Ecstasy is the street name for 3,4-methlyenedioxymethamphetamine (MDMA). *Belladonna* ingestion, such as deadly nightshade, results in an anticholinergic toxidrome. Spice is the street name for a synthetic cannabinoid receptor agonist. Mephedrone is a synthetic cathinone.

Further reading

Bateman D, et al. *Oxford Desk Reference: Toxicology*. Oxford University Press, 2014.

Smith S, Scarth E. *Drugs in Anaesthesia and Intensive Care*, 5th edition. Oxford University Press, 2016. Atropine.

Single Best Answers

1. D

While all of the options are important elements within this patient's management, the primary concern is to ensure patient and staff safety which may include induction of anaesthesia, intubation, ventilation, and continued sedation on intensive care. If the patient lacks capacity, then he should be treated in his 'best interests' in this emergency scenario. Collecting urine for a rapid drug screen is an important subsequent step, although if this man has ingested a synthetic cannabinoid receptor agonist such as 'spice', this would not be routinely detected on current urine drug screens. A serum blood sample taken as soon as is practically possible is a sensible step to take with a request to the local pathology department to store the sample as it may need to be sent off to a tertiary toxicology centre in due course. The possibility of an acute intracranial event should always be considered in any individual with acute neurological symptoms. Obtaining a collateral history, if possible, can often lead to invaluable information in making a diagnosis.

Further reading

Bateman D, et al. *Oxford Desk Reference: Toxicology*. Oxford University Press, 2014.

2. C

Psilocybin (derived from *Psilocybe* species) does cause abdominal pain and vomiting, but in addition is usually associated with neuropsychiatric symptoms typically occurring within 20–240 minutes following ingestion. Amatoxin ingestion (derived from *Amanita* species) could fit with the symptom complex described but seizure activity is not a feature. *Gyromitra* species produce gyromitrin which undergoes hydrolysis to a gamma-aminobutyric acid (GABA) inhibitor, monomethylhydrazine, which when metabolized further results in hepatic damage. Coprine ingestion (derived from *Coprinus* species) causes a disulfiram-like reaction when ingested with ethanol. *Orellanine* species may result in renal failure but typically seven days following ingestion.

Further reading

Bateman D, et al. *Oxford Desk Reference: Toxicology*. Oxford University Press, 2014.

3. E

Cholinergic and opioid ingestion result in miosis. Hallucinogenic agents such as LSD cause mydriasis and agitation but are not associated with seizure activity. Anticholinergic agents are not associated with seizures. Sympathomimetic agents, such as synthetic cathinones and synthetic cannabinoids, cause the pattern of clinical features described.

Further reading

Bateman D, et al. *Oxford Desk Reference: Toxicology*. Oxford University Press, 2014.

Dignam G, Bigham C. Novel psychoactive substances: a practical approach to dealing with toxicity from legal highs. *BJA Education*, 2017;17(5):172–177.

Smith S, Scarth E. *Drugs in Anaesthesia and Intensive Care*, 5th edition. Oxford University Press, 2016. Atropine, Morphine.

4. C

Exposure to any of the agents may result in the clinical features described. Phosgene, ammonia, and sulphuric acid exposure may cause identical symptoms and should be included in the differential diagnosis. However, following public order disturbance it is most likely that the patients have been exposed to chlorobenzylidenemalononitrile or 'CS' spray, commonly known as 'tear gas'. UK police forces use a 5% w/v CS gas spray with an organic solvent so that it can be aerosolized as the agent itself is a solid at room temperature. Chloroacetophenone (CN) is a less potent lachrymator, has a slower onset time yet is associated with greater toxicity than CS gas so its use has been largely superseded by CS. CN is the principal agent in mace.

Further reading

Bateman D, et al. *Oxford Desk Reference: Toxicology*. Oxford University Press, 2014.

5. A

Malignant neuroleptic syndrome is typically associated with the chronic use of antipsychotic agents, of which there is no history suggestive of their use. Phaeochromocytoma, while a possible diagnosis, seems unlikely, especially given the reduced GCS. Malignant hyperpyrexia should be considered if suxamethonium (a depolarizing muscle relaxant) was used to facilitate tracheal intubation but most pre-hospital specialists would use rocuronium (a non-depolarizing muscle relaxant). Suxamethonium can be a trigger for malignant hyperpyrexia, but it is not associated with non-depolarizing agent use. Amphetamine usage would fit the clinical features described. Heat stroke, while a possible diagnosis, seems unlikely in the context of seizure activity.

Further reading

Bateman D, et al. *Oxford Desk Reference: Toxicology*. Oxford University Press, 2014.

Smith S, Scarth E. *Drugs in Anaesthesia and Intensive Care*, 5th edition. Oxford University Press, 2016. Dantrolene, Suxamethonium.

6. E

The most rapid form of detection will be the signs and symptom complexes of the victims of the attack. Detection equipment will take time to be deployed and used. Chemical detection paper uses a colour change to determine liquid nerve agents. Fourier-transform infrared spectroscopy can be used in a hand-held device which contains a molecular database of agents for comparison to the suspected agent. Raman spectrometers can also be used in portable devices. Gas chromatography-mass spectroscopy is the most accurate technology available to detect single or multiple agents.

Further reading

Bateman D, et al. *Oxford Desk Reference: Toxicology*. Oxford University Press, 2014.

7. C

Americium is excreted from the body within a few days and little enters the bloodstream. Plutonium is poorly absorbed from the gastrointestinal (GI) tract. Polonium emits a very high number of alpha particles. Due to this high alpha decay, it emits a high amount of radiation. Thorium has low radioactivity. Uranium is excreted within a few days following ingestion.

Further reading

Bateman D, et al. *Oxford Desk Reference: Toxicology*. Oxford University Press, 2014.

Index

For the benefit of digital users, indexed terms that span two pages (e.g., 52–53) may, on occasion, appear on only one of those pages.
Tables are indicated by *t* following the page number